Health Security Intelligence

The book takes a multi-disciplinary approach to explore the role national security intelligence agencies played in supporting national governments' response to COVID-19.

Spanning the 'Five Eyes' intelligence countries (UK, USA, Canada, Australia and New Zealand), this book offers the first cross-comparative analysis of what intelligence agencies need to focus on in responding more effectively to future emerging health and biological security threats risks and hazards post-COVID-19. The volume addresses three principal issues. First, it investigates what roles the Five Eyes intelligence communities played (along with other key stakeholders, such as public health agencies) in managing the COVID-19 pandemic. Second, it assesses the challenges of and lessons learnt from these intelligence communities' engagement in managing aspects of the pandemic. Third, it explores how the Five Eyes might play more effective roles in managing future health security threats and risks, whether those are intentional (bioterrorism and bio crimes), accidental (laboratory releases) or unintentional (pandemics) in origin. Overall, this book offers a coherent and holistic research agenda that seeks to improve understanding about the role of national security intelligence in managing health security threats and risks post-COVID-19.

This book will be of much interest to students of intelligence studies, health security, public health and International Relations.

Patrick F. Walsh is a Professor of Intelligence and Security Studies at Charles Sturt University, Australia. He is a former intelligence analyst who has worked in Australian national security and law enforcement agencies. He has written multiple books and research articles on intelligence capability issues, including related to health and biological security.

Studies in Intelligence

General Editors: Richard J. Aldrich, Claudia Hillebrand and Christopher Andrew

For more information about this series, please visit: www.routledge.com/Studies-in-Intelligence/book-series/SE0788

Health Security Intelligence

Managing Emerging Threats and Risks in a
Post-Covid World

Edited by Patrick F. Walsh

Routledge
Taylor & Francis Group

LONDON AND NEW YORK

First published 2025
by Routledge
4 Park Square, Milton Park, Abingdon, Oxon OX14 4RN

and by Routledge
605 Third Avenue, New York, NY 10158

Routledge is an imprint of the Taylor & Francis Group, an informa business

British Library Cataloguing-in-Publication Data
A catalogue record for this book is available from the British Library

ISBN: 978-1-032-37144-3 (hbk)
ISBN: 978-1-032-37145-0 (pbk)
ISBN: 978-1-003-33551-1 (ebk)

DOI: 10.4324/9781003335511

Typeset in Times New Roman
by Newgen Publishing UK

Contents

Figures

Contributors

Ausma Bernot is a Lecturer in Criminology at the School of Criminology and Criminal Justice, Griffith University, Australia. Her work is focused on surveillance and technology governance.

Gemma Bowsher co-leads on global health security programs at the Centre for Conflict and Health Research at Kings College London. She is a social scientist and physician and her work focuses on the interface of health security, CBRN and cyber threats in complex settings, particularly those experiencing conflict.

Erik Dahl is Associate Professor of National Security affairs at the Naval Postgraduate School in Monterey, California, USA. He is a retired U.S Naval Intelligence officer, and former chair of the Intelligence Studies Section of the International Studies Association.

Jennifer Hunt is a Senior Lecturer in Cyber and Security Studies at Macquarie University, Sydney, Australia, specializing in cyber conflict and information warfare.

Filippa Lentzos is a Reader (Associate Professor) in Science & International Security, with a joint appointment in the Department of War Studies and in the Department of Global Health & Social Medicine at Kings College London.

Seumas Miller is Professor of Philosophy at Charles Sturt University, Australia and Distinguished Research Fellow at the University of Oxford.

David Skillicorn is a Professor currently working in the School of Computing for Queens University. He also works as an Adjunct Professor in the Mathematics and Computer Science Department of the Royal Military College, Canada.

Kathleen M. Vogel is a Professor at the School for the Future of Innovation in Society and Senior Global Futures Scientist. Global Futures Laboratory at Arizona State University, USA.

Patrick F. Walsh is a Professor of Intelligence and Security Studies at Charles Sturt University, Australia. He is a former intelligence analyst who has worked in Australian national security and law enforcement agencies.

Acknowledgements

This research and the open access publication of the manuscript was supported by funding from two research grants. In particular, Patrick F. Walsh (the editor) and Professor Seumas Miller gratefully acknowledge funding from the Australian Research Council Discovery Grant DP180103439, Intelligence and National Security: Ethics, Efficacy and Accountability. Professor Seumas Miller gratefully acknowledges funding from the European Research Council Advanced Grant (GTCMR: 670172), Global Terrorism and Collective Responsibility: Redesigning Military, Police and intelligence Institutions in Liberal Democracies. Patrick F. Walsh also thanks Charles Sturt University's one-year funding for a post-doctoral fellow (Dr Ausma Bernot) from its Contemporary Threats to Australian Security program which supported this publication. Lastly, a big heartfelt thanks to all the excellent contributors to this volume for your excellent insights and commitment to this project.

Part I

Health Security Intelligence and COVID-19

1 Introduction

Patrick F. Walsh

Objectives and Overview

According to the World Health Organization (WHO), reporting from 5 January 2020 to 3 March 2024, the total (cumulative) number of global COVID-19 cases is estimated to be over 774 million infections with 7 million deaths.[1] Beyond the significant loss of life lies profound global economic, political, and social changes. Its impacts remain poorly understood even four years since the onset of the pandemic and will likely affect nations for generations. In many liberal democracies, including the 'Five Eyes' countries (United States, United Kingdom, Australia, Canada and New Zealand) there has been increasing commentary that the political, economic, social and of course public health impacts of the COVID-19 pandemic are having, and will continue to have, national security implications.

However, the extent to which health security events regardless of their origin (intentional malicious acts or natural/accidental) are national security threats remains contested by differing academic and practitioner perspectives. These debates are not new, though COVID-19 brings them back into the spotlight. In this book the editor, contributors and other scholars whose work is cited in it, increasingly hold the view that health security threats and risks, such as pandemics, do have national security implications (Wilson 2017, Wilson et al. 2013; Dahl 2023; Walsh 2018; 2020a, 586–602; Walsh 2020b; Wark 2020; 2021; Bowsher et al. 2020: 1–9; Lentzos, Goodman and Wilson 2020, 465–76). As noted, however, such a view is not universal. Moreover, the research agendas of health security scholars, who have assessed the national security implications of health threats and risks have not always grabbed the attention of policy makers or intelligence studies scholars. Despite an inconsistent focus and understanding of the national security dimensions of health threats/risks since 9/11, the COVID-19 pandemic provides an opportunity for a renewed attention by policy makers on these issues. It is unclear, however, whether the same level of policy maker focus demonstrated during the acute phase of the COVID-19 crisis will remain in the current post-emergency phase of the pandemic. Already, evidence suggests this is less likely. Additionally, can we expect now any broader policy reforms that will eventually translate into paradigmatic changes in how 'Five Eyes' intelligence communities perceive and understand health security issues four years since the pandemic started in the current post-emergency phase?

DOI: 10.4324/9781003335511-2

Will our ICs view them (health security issues) as being in the same vein as other core and traditional national security threats/risks such as great power competition or terrorism? Or alternatively, as the international community continues to shift into a post-COVID-19 world, will intelligence agencies revert back to playing only a marginal or supportive role in dealing with future pandemics? The terrorist attacks on the United States (September 11, 2001) resulted in major reforms to how the U.S. intelligence community (U.S. IC) and its allies responded to a new evolution in global terrorism. Will the existential nature of COVID-19 usher in similar profound reforms to 'Five Eyes' intelligence communities that will allow them to play a more significant role in detecting, preventing and managing future health security threats, risks and hazards? Time will tell. Already though, debates are underway by scholars and policy makers about the role played by national security intelligence agencies during COVID-19 and whether they were effective – as well as what resources and capabilities 'Five Eyes' ICs should be harnessed for future pandemics (Walsh et al. 2023, 1095–1111). For example, debates are developing about whether sub-optimal global and national warning systems designed to warn nations about the emerging COVID-19 pandemic represents another example of intelligence failure like the events of 9/11 (Dahl 2023; Gressang and Wirtz 2021). There has also been increasing discussion about the specific roles 'Five Eyes' intelligence agencies have played. Discussions have included how some intelligence agencies have supported public health contact tracing and health orders, detecting public health misinformation and assessing COVID-19 origins during the pandemic (Walsh et al. 2023, 1095–1111). Similarly, COVID-19 has facilitated several biocybersecurity attacks against global pharmaceuticals and underscored several vulnerabilities in critical health infrastructure and supply chains.[2] For example, the malicious cyber hacking of big pharmaceuticals such as Pfizer BioNTech to steal IP related to mRNA vaccines during COVID-19 can impact on the political, health, economic and social wellbeing of countries (Walsh 2022, 335–355). Additionally, such state-sponsored and non-state actor attacks on biotechnology industries can impact scientific collaboration. A reduced willingness by countries to share scientific data could in turn potentially result in delays in scientific discoveries that harm the health of patients (Walsh 2022, 335–355).

COVID-19 is the result of several other strategic drivers that are worsening globally and likely will continue to have national security implications for many states. A combination of variables including climate change, globalisation and ecological degradation that brings animals carrying novel infections closer to humans – resulting in new zoonotic diseases. This means that consequential non-routine disease outbreaks are likely to be more common in the future (Frutos et al. 2020; Mallapaty 2020; Murray 2020). At the same time, rapid changes in synthetic biology, biotechnology and the digitisation of bioprocessing in the global bioeconomy while opening new industries and beneficial products in agriculture, pharmaceuticals and energy provide opportunities for these to be exploited by state and non-state actors.

This book explores all these health security debates – some of which extend back several decades prior to COVID-19 and others which have become strident recently due to the COVID-19 pandemic. The book seeks to contribute to these debates by addressing three critical aims. First, it investigates what roles 'Five Eyes' intelligence communities played (along with other key stakeholders such as public health agencies) in managing COVID-19. Second, it assesses the challenges and lessons learnt for 'Five Eyes' intelligence communities in how they have engaged in managing aspects of the COVID-19 pandemic? Thirdly, how may 'Five Eyes' intelligence communities play more effective roles in managing future health security threats and risks – whether these are intentional (bioterrorism and bio crimes), accidental (accidental laboratory releases) or unintentional (pandemics) in origin.

Given the existential nature of COVID-19 and other recent pandemics, it is critical that these questions are investigated in a timely fashion. An increasing number of complex health security threats, risks and hazards will likely emerge that can have significant impact on the economic, social and health wellbeing of nations in the next few decades. As with COVID-19, the assessment of both the likelihood and consequences of threats/risks/hazards and the ability by nations to prevent, disrupt and mitigate them will require even more effective whole of society responses and in most cases the aggressive pursuit of public–private partnerships than has been the case before. This will mean the ability of all levers of government including public health authorities, national security intelligence agencies and the private sector being able to work together in more coordinated and effective ways to manage health security threats that have the potential to impact on all aspects of society. However, what is not understood sufficiently is what role both strategically and operationally should intelligence communities play in a world that presents a range of potential yet complex health security threats, risks and hazards? What unique value add can the 'Five Eyes' intelligence communities offer to public health authorities and other responders as part of an all-hazards and whole of society approach to managing such threats, risks and hazards? What are the boundaries between what resources and capabilities our intelligence agencies can bring to bear in managing health security threats and risks; and what is the role of other public and private stakeholders?

As many of the health security threats/risks/hazards post COVID-19 become more complex, clearer, more evidenced based decisions will need to be made by policy makers, our intelligence communities and other health security stakeholders about what role ICs can usefully play in preventing, disrupting and managing health security threats/risks/hazards post COVID. This book fills a major gap in the intelligence studies literature about what role 'Five Eyes' intelligence enterprises should play in supporting policy makers, researchers, the public and private health sector, in understanding health security threats/risks in a post-COVID-19 world. Given the significant loss of life, economic and social damages wrought by this pandemic, should such an impactful event change how national security intelligence agencies play a role in the strategic and operational management of health security threats, risks and hazards in the future? The contributors to this edited volume believe so, and this book provides insights into how 'Five Eyes' intelligence communities can play a larger collaborative role in dealing with future health security threats, risks and hazards. While sometimes the 'fog' of a crisis makes it difficult for policy makers and practitioners to reflect immediately on the lessons to be learnt – now four years post-pandemic it is timely to develop better knowledge, processes and capabilities across the health security intelligence enterprise in order to respond more effectively to likely future threats, risks and hazards.

This edited collection brings together a multi-disciplinary approach to understanding emerging health security threats and hazards. It investigates the role 'Five Eyes' intelligence partners could play (singly and collectively) in managing them post COVID-19. In particular, the volume is a fusion of perspectives from experts with extensive backgrounds in national security intelligence, and other fields including but not limited to biodefence, public health, ethics, computer science, medicine, biotechnology, and science and technology – to better understand emerging health security threats/risks/hazards and to determine the role national security intelligence could play in managing them. Additionally, the volume synthesises perspectives from academic, government and private industry sources.

As noted earlier, this book explores three aims. First, it will assess how the national security intelligence enterprises in 'Five Eyes' countries played a role in responding to health security threats and risks in the immediate period leading up to and including the COVID-19 pandemic commencing in 2019. Second, and reflecting on the background provided in the book's first section, it investigates what key challenges exist in managing health security threats/risks/hazards for 'Five Eyes' national security intelligence enterprises, in collaboration with the public health, research community and private sector? Third, and reflecting on these challenges, the book explores what opportunities exist for national security intelligence agencies in collaboration with other stakeholders to better manage health security threats and risks post-COVID-19? In summary, the book will address four key objectives:

1 Understand and define key contested terminology such as national security intelligence, health security, health security intelligence, biosecurity and intelligence failure.
2 Understand the context of how national security intelligence agencies across the 'Five Eyes' became involved in responding to the COVID-19 pandemic.
3 Assess (post-COVID-19) the key challenges in managing future pandemics and other health security threats and risks for national security intelligence agencies, public health, the research community and the private sector?
4 Identify opportunities for national security intelligence agencies, public health, the research community and the private sector to better mitigate health security threats and risks post-COVID-19.

The Audience

Given the multi-disciplinary approach taken, we believe it will be useful to researchers, policy-makers and practitioners, who have a stake in understanding, preventing and managing emerging health security threats, risks and hazards post-COVID-19. The primary audience will be those working in 'Five Eyes' intelligence communities (and other liberal democracies), who seek to improve capabilities in order to more effectively support other public health, scientists and first responders in managing health security threats, risks and hazards. However, we also see this volume as being useful for a range of other stakeholders (e.g., public health, global health officials, researchers and the private sector), who need a greater understanding of how 'Five Eyes' intelligence communities might play more effective roles in the detection, prevention, warning and response to health security threats and risks. A third audience for the book, we hope, will be scholars, who do research in health security intelligence capability reform issues as well as others outside of the intelligence studies discipline, who are interested in health security areas. Finally, through this volume we seek to engage students contemplating higher degrees and encourage them to take up their own research projects on health security intelligence issues.

The Book's Points of Difference

As discussed above, this book's editor and contributors have published frequently on health security topics (e.g., Walsh 2016, 2018, 2020a, 2021; 2023; Dahl 2023; Goodman, Wilson and Lentzos 2021; Bowsher et al. 2020, Bowsher and Sullivan 2021; Miller and Smith 2021; Henscke et al. 2024) in recent years. However, what has been missing is a comprehensive book on health security *intelligence* which brings together all relevant aspects of health security intelligence (e.g., collection, analysis, policy, capability gaps, technology, ethics and collaboration) in one volume and shows how they are connected for a national security intelligence, public health, research and private sector scholarly and practitioner audience. While some excellent works have been recently published on health security and health security intelligence issues (see, for example, Dahl 2023; West et al. 2021) the intelligence studies literature has not focused deeply or sufficiently on health security intelligence. And, traditionally, what health security intelligence-related topics (e.g., pandemics, CBRN/WMD, bioterrorism, biosecurity, biosafety amongst others) are covered have generally been dealt with through the narrower prisms of biodefence or global health (Walsh 2018). Such approaches restrict the focus, understanding and solutions down to a siloed 'biodefence' or 'public health' threat/risk-centric approach – not ones that are sufficiently multi-disciplinary or necessarily fully one-health in perspective. While several pre-COVID-19 volumes include health security-related material, they are treated through a biodefense prism with a threat agent (state or non-state actor) weaponing a biological agent (Singh and Kuhn 2019; Burnette 2013; Bombardt 2000). In particular, the literature and government investments has been on attribution of intentional health threats/risks while leaving significant knowledge gaps in other health security capabilities such as global monitoring. As COVID-19 has demonstrated, a bias by practitioners and in the literature on intentional attribution has been problematic as a final accurate assessment on attribution can take a long time to resolve after a health security crisis such as a pandemic (natural, accidental or intentional) has occurred. This book will discuss the importance of threat actors and attribution, but through a broader national security and one health framework context that also examines the security, health, social and broader economic risks posed by threat actors.

The first point of innovation, therefore, is a book that investigates in depth and breadth all aspects of health security intelligence from a multi-disciplinary perspective. The book will bring together in the one place health security perspectives from intelligence studies scholars, medicine, computer science, biodefence, biotechnology, synthetic biology and ethics to define how national security intelligence agencies, public health, research and the private sector can work together on health security threats and risks. While the key focus is on how 'Five Eyes' intelligence enterprises might play a more strategically and operationally engaged role in health security threats, risks and hazards post-COVID-19, we will demonstrate how emerging health security threats and risks will demand national security agencies work more collaboratively with a suite of multi-disciplinary, public and private sector actors. Additionally, although the COVID-19 pandemic has recently become a catalyst for a growing body of research and policy maker attention on various aspects of health security intelligence, particularly early warning failure (Dahl 2023; Cho 2020; G20 2021; GPHIN Review 2021; Wark 2021; Mehta 2020), what is needed is the development of a more coherent research and policy agenda about the role of national security intelligence in the broader health security intelligence field and vice versa. This research agenda must include the investigation of a broader range of health security threats, risks and hazards. Such an agenda would include not only the role national security intelligence agencies should play in managing future pandemics, but also a range of other emerging health security threats, risks and hazards emerging via animal health, synthetic biology, biotechnology and the digitisation of biology. Hence this book will, for the first time, map a coherent and holistic research agenda (see Chapters 8 and 10) that seeks a common understanding about the role of national security intelligence in managing health security threats, risks and hazards post-COVID-19.

A second point of innovation is the cross-comparative (examining selected 'Five Eyes' alliance countries) focus of the book – including exploring what health security intelligence role selected national security agencies played in these countries during COVID-19. Each chapter will, to the extent possible, draw on case examples and knowledge across 'Five Eyes' countries when addressing key chapter themes. This will provide a rich contextual analysis of health security intelligence themes, issues and help identify where good practice resides across both the national security, health and disciplines with relevant stakeholders.

There are naturally currently limitations to how comprehensive the analysis can be of the roles played by all 'Five Eyes' intelligence agencies during COVID-19. Much of this type of information remains restricted. However, four years post the emergence of the pandemic, scholars – through access to government reporting, inquiries and research – are getting better knowledge of what roles particular intelligence agencies played in supporting governments through the pandemic. This book will build on that available knowledge, particularly in providing a normative approach to how 'Five Eyes' intelligence agencies ought to improve their post-COVID-19 health security intelligence capabilities.

Book Structure

In order to address the four research objectives, this collection is divided into three sections with ten chapters. The first section, 'Health Security Intelligence and COVID-19', provides the theoretical and contextual foundations and comprises two chapters. Chapter 1 (this chapter) by the editor introduces the aims, objectives and structure of the volume. In Chapter 2 ('Framing National Security and Health Security Intelligence'), Erik Dahl explores the theoretical, policy and practitioner debates surrounding key terminology used throughout the book including intelligence, national security intelligence, intelligence failure, health security, and health security intelligence. Other key themes in Dahl's chapter are collection methodologies, and securitisation of health. Dahl concludes by arguing COVID-19 represented an intelligence failure. This conclusion is linked to more fundamental questions about whether intelligence agencies had been providing sufficient warning and if decision-makers acted appropriately on the intelligence provided. Intelligence failure is a theme returned to in Chapter 10 ('Conclusion').

Section 2, 'Challenges in Managing Health Security Threats, Risks and Hazards', consists of two chapters. Chapter 3 ('Political Engagement') by Patrick F. Walsh and Ausma Bernot identifies thematically several key barriers including: political, institutional, cultural, factors that have constrained the role many 'Five Eyes' intelligence agencies played in dealing with major health security threats and risks such as COVID-19. The chapter argues that these constraining factors are not new, but rather are long-standing, stretching back to 9/11 and earlier. The chapter surveys how different administrations in the United Kingdom and the United States have shaped the policy framework for WMD, biodefence and health security emergencies from post-World War Two up to COVID-19. It examines how political rhetoric and disengagement has historically not consistently translated into a coordinated investment by 'Five Eyes' governments in key areas of health security including in effective preparedness, governance, threat assessment and international coordination.

Chapter 4, 'Disinformation: The COVID-19 Pandemic and Beyond', by Jennifer Hunt focuses on the role of disinformation, including cyber-enabled disinformation during COVID-19 and its long-term implications in the current post-acute pandemic period. The chapter explores in detail how disinformation propagated by state actors, religious/ideologically motivated terrorists and hosts of other issue motivated groups coalesced around several categories. These categories included: the origins of COVID-19, the pandemic's severity, and the effectiveness or otherwise of government responses. Hunt shows how disinformation was most effective when spread by groups (e.g., military, law enforcement and officers of the courts) with a high degree of trust particularly in the United States. Chapter 4 underscores how, during COVID-19, disinformation became a kind of pollution and concludes with insights from social science research in psychology, political science and communication studies to support the design of counter health security related disinformation narratives. Also discussed is the role of new AI tools alongside enhanced efforts in regulation, education and enforcement to counter public health misinformation/disinformation and conspiracy theories into the future. What role national security intelligence agencies should play in countering disinformation campaigns is a theme discussed further in Chapter 10 ('Conclusion').

Section 3, 'Improving Health Security Threat and Risk Mitigation', consists of six chapters. Each chapter focuses thematically on areas where 'Five Eyes' intelligence communities can make enhanced investments in planning, resources, knowledge, workforce and research in their health security intelligence capabilities post-COVID-19. In Chapter 5 ('Building Better Health Security Intelligence Strategies Post COVID-19'), Gemma Bowsher, reflecting on the many challenges arising out of COVID-19 outlined in Sections 1 and 2 for 'Five Eyes' countries, underscores the need for more effective strategic and operational responses to respond to emerging health security threats and risks. Bowsher builds on the political and institutional challenges identified in Chapter 3 by Walsh and Bernot leading up to COVID-19. The chapter explores how, during COVID-19, similar capability constraints identified in Chapter 3 impacted the advancement of health security intelligence management goals of individual 'Five Eyes' nations and on the ability of the alliance to integrate intelligence approaches for mutual benefit. As the first chapter in Section 3, Bowsher's chapter takes a macro perspective on how individual and collective 'Five Eyes' countries might improve their intelligence capabilities, along with public health and other key stakeholders to deliver improved integrated domestic and international responses to health security emergencies. Bowsher argues that now in the post-emergency period of COVID-19, there is some evidence of 'Five Eyes' intelligence communities working more effectively on health security, for example on the issue of the origins of the pandemic and how national security approaches to early warning might inform the development of more robust disease early warning systems used by WHO and national public health institutions which have traditionally relied on epidemiological intelligence. Such achievements need to be expanded on going forward and Bowsher provides several examples of how particular strategies and institutional arrangements within and across 'Five Eyes 'alliance could provide foundations for innovation and growth in health security intelligence capabilities in the future.

Following the broader road map for developing more effective 'Five Eyes' intelligence capabilities provided in Chapter 5, Chapters 6 to 9 drill down in specific areas relevant to improving 'Five Eyes' health security intelligence threats in the current post-emergency COVID-19 period. In Chapter 6 ('Improving Health Security Intelligence Warning Systems'), David Skillicorn, from a computer science and machine learning perspective, explores whether we can really have more robust health security intelligence warning systems within and across 'Five Eyes' countries. Several earlier chapters and Miller's discussion in the following chapter (Chapter 7 'Biosecurity, National Security Intelligence and Ethics') have already raised other challenges (e.g., epidemiological, political, policy and ethical) in designing health security intelligence warning systems in the past leading up to COVID-19. Chapter 6 asks whether, from a technical perspective, proactive rather than reactive early warning is possible? Skillicorn explores how should we assess the value of indicators used for warning and shows how the significance of indicator values depends on a range of complex principles including the provenance, relationship of indicators to semantics, context and rates of change. Skillicorn poses several other fundamental questions that require careful reflection in the development of any meaningful health security intelligence warning systems, particularly how a judgement of 'significance' is not made based on a single set of indicators in isolation, nor even the historical record of a single indicator, but is instead based on the collective pattern of all indicators over all the historical records. Chapter 6 concludes with a discussion on the real technical challenges that still remain in building better health security intelligence warning systems that can 'warn' or detect inherently rare events. The chapter offers suggestions on how particular techniques such as neural network-based clustering algorithms or a Bayesian approach might help improve anomaly detection, though Skillicorn concludes more research is needed on how to select good indicators as well as resolving other non-technical issues such as convincing governments to pay for their collection and getting warning products to multiple stakeholders across the health security intelligence enterprise.

In Chapter 7 ('Biosecurity, National Security Intelligence and Ethics'), Seumas Miller assesses the ethical challenges for public health, security and law enforcement officials accessing diverse data sets (e.g., social media and health data) to mitigate against various biosecurity and broader health security threats and risks. Miller first examines several areas of biosecurity (e.g. bio-bank and data base security, pandemics and dual use problems) and via a detail conceptual analysis identifies the moral problems both associated with threat actors who might exploit them, but also the ethical principles and challenges faced by national security intelligence agencies in collecting and analysing 'bio-data' and other health data in order to thwart malevolent activities of bad actors. In Chapter 8 '(Improving the Health Security Intelligence Workforce and Research Agenda') Kathleen Vogel explores two key related strands critical to the success in building health security intelligence capabilities across the 'Five Eyes' countries-workforce planning and the development of impactful research agendas that build future capabilities. Vogel asks given the now worldwide retirement of bio-weapons experts from most 'Five Eyes' intelligence communities, how do we prepare the current and next generation of intelligence collectors, analysts and the IC leadership to develop skills, knowledge, and competencies across the range of health security related disciplines? Vogel's chapter highlights the complexities underpinning how 'Five Eyes' intelligence communities should plan for a skilled workforce in a multi-disciplinary area such as health security. In many of our 'Five Eyes' intelligence agencies, particularly within the intelligence analyst's sections, we have seen debates about whether 'generalist' analysts are more cost-effective and flexible rather than subject matter experts because the former can at least be more flexibly redeployed as new 'issues of the day' arise. But this approach clearly has its downsides in the ability for analysts to deeply understand complex issues around public health, bio-defence, molecular biology or biotechnology where there may be security concerns. It is also obvious that intelligence communities cannot feasibly build deep expertise in the fields of medicine, public health and the biological. As the 2021 publicly released US Office of Director of National Intelligence report on the origins of SARS-COV-2 shows, with complex health and biological security issues such as this, our intelligence communities will always need to rely on external scientific and technical expertise. This won't change in the future, but Vogel's chapters and others in the book make the point that intelligence analysts still need expertise in the interpretation of scientific material and how it relates to other sources of intelligence collected. So, the question remains going forward, how do 'Five Eyes' intelligence communities build this expertise in ways that build a corporate repository of knowledge on health security intelligence issues inside the community yet are cost effective and still allow analysts to seek advice from experts outside of the national security enterprise.

In the second half of Chapter 8, Vogel pivots and asks how new knowledge can be generated from future health security intelligence related research? The chapter concludes by introducing the key components of a health security research agenda which identifies and prioritises areas where new health security knowledge and practice can improve the workforce for both 'Five Eyes' intelligence communities and stakeholders. Research priorities will also be returned to in Chapter 10 ('Conclusion'). In Chapter 9 ('Managing Health Security Threats at the Multilateral Level'), Filippa Lentzos explores several critical themes around the role of multilateral institutions such the WHO, and other global countermeasures and compliance mechanisms aimed at preventing, disrupting and mitigating against emerging health security threats, risks and hazards beyond COVID-19. Lentzos frames her discussion about the need for stronger multilateral action on future health security emergencies on the foundation of rising risks in the natural outbreaks from zoonotic transmissions, the risks of lab accidents with the rise of gain of function experiments – and the expansion of science and technology knowledge increasing the potential rise in bioweapons from hostile actors. Lentzos shows how the WHO-led multilateral efforts to investigate the origins of COVID-19 became politicised, lacking transparency with incomplete results. In particular, a lack of access of data and biological samples in China by non- Chinese nationals on the Joint WHO–China team fuelled further speculation and division in 'Five Eyes' capitals, particularly Washington DC, about the origins of COVID-19. Speculation arose in the Trump Administration and some members of Congress that the COVID-19 pandemic was more likely than not the result of a research-related incident. As noted in earlier chapters, it was during this politicised background that the incoming Biden Administration tasked the US IC to shed light on whether COVID-19 origins were intentional, natural or accidental. While discounting early that it was a bioweapon, the US intelligence community remains split between a 'lab leak' or natural event scenario. There are clearly lessons to be learnt from the COVID-19 origins incident about how to improve multilateral monitoring and investigations of ambiguous health security threats, risks and hazards. Lentzos outlines in detail a proposal for investigating ambiguous origin investigations in the future facilitated through an investigative body via WHO and its International Health Regulations. This public health rather than security approach might gain more traction from a politically fractured international community where current proposals to establish a new multilaterally agreed treaty /pandemic agreement for future preparedness and response appears to be in jeopardy. Chapter 12 ('Conclusion') summarises key themes identified in each chapter with a view to identifying critical next policy, institutional and research steps for developing health security intelligence knowledge in both national security, public and animal health, and the research and private sector communities. The final chapter has three objectives. First, to revisit key themes identified in the book. Second, it will propose institutional and policy reforms that may help better prepare both 'Five Eyes' countries and stakeholders for the next inevitable health security threat, risk or hazard. Finally, it suggests a research agenda for health security intelligence to engage both the 'Five Eyes' intelligence community and key public and private stakeholders.

Notes

1 These figures are obviously significantly underestimated. See WHO Coronavirus (COVID-19) Dashboard: https://data.who.int/dashboards/covid19/cases
2 Bio-cybersecurity, or as its sometimes also referred to as 'cyber-biosecurity', is a new field that seeks to protect digitalised biological and health data to safeguard the individual, public, health care infrastructure and the development of biotechnological innovation.

References

Bombardt, J. (2000). *Contagious Disease Dynamics for Biological Warfare and Bioterrorism Casualty Assessments*. US Department of Defense.

Bowsher, G., Bernard, R., & Sullivan, R. (2020). A Health Intelligence Framework for Pandemic Response: Lessons from the UK Experience of COVID-19. *Health Security*, *18*(6), 1–9.

Bowsher, G., & Sullivan, R. (2021). Why We Need an Intelligence-Led Approach to Pandemics: Supporting Science and Public Health During COVID-19 and Beyond. *Journal of the Royal Society of the Medicine*, *114*(1), 12–14.

Burnette, R. (Ed.) (2013). *Biosecurity Understanding, Assessing, and Preventing the Threat*. Wiley.

Cho, A. (2020). Artificial Intelligence Systems Aim to Sniff Out Signs of COVID 19 Outbreaks. *Science*, *368*, 810–811. doi:10.1126/science.368.6493.810

Dahl, E. J. (2023). *The COVID-19 Intelligence Failure: Why Warning Was Not Enough*. Georgetown University Press.

Frutos, R., Lopez Roig, M., Serra-Cobo, J., & Devaux, C. A. (2020). COVID-19: The Conjunction of Events Leading to the Coronavirus Pandemic and Lessons to Learn for Future Threats. *Frontiers in Medicine*, *7*(223), doi:10.3389/fmed.2020.00223

G20 (2021). *A Global Deal for Our Pandemic Age*. G20.

Goodman, M. S., Wilson, J. M., & Lentzos, F. (Eds.) (2021). *Health Security Intelligence*. Routledge.

GPHIN External Review Panel (2021). *Independent Review of Canada's GPHIN*. Ottawa. www.canada.ca/en/public-health/corporate/mandate/about-agency/external-advisory-bodies/list/independent-review-global-public-health-intelligence-network/interim-rep ort.html

Gressang, D. S., & Wirtz, J. J. (2021). Rethinking Warning: Intelligence, Novel Events, and the COVID-19 Pandemic. *International Journal of Intelligence and Counterintelligence*, *35*(1), 131–146. doi:10.1080/08850607.2021.1913023

Henschke, A., Miller, S., Alexandra, A., Walsh, P. F., & Bradbury, R. (2024). *The Ethics of National Security Intelligence Institutions: Theory and Applications* (p. 249). Taylor & Francis.

Lentzos, F., Goodman, M. S., & Wilson, J. M. (2020). Health Security Intelligence: Engaging Across Disciplines and Sectors. *Intelligence and National Security*, *35*(4), 465–476.

Magid, A., Gesser-Edelsburg, A., & Green, M. S. (2018). The Role of Informal Digital Surveillance Systems Before, During and After Infectious Disease Outbreaks: A Critical Analysis. In Radosavljevic, V., Banjari, I., & Belojevic, G. (eds.), *Defence Against Bioterrorism: Methods for Prevention and Control* (pp. 189–201). Springer. https://doi. org/10.1007/978-94-024-1263-5_14

Mallapaty, S. (2020). Scientists Call for Pandemic Investigations to Focus on Wildlife Trade. *Nature*, *583*, 344.

Mehta, M. C., Katz, I. T., & Jha, A. K. (2020). Transforming Global Health with AI. *New England Journal of Medicine*, *382*(9), 791–793. doi:10.1056/NEJMp1912079

Miller, S., & Smith, M. (2021). Ethics, Public Health and Technology Responses to COVID-19. *Bioethics*, *35*(4), 366–371.

Murray, K. A., Escobar, L. E., Lowe, R., Rocklöv, J., Semenza, J. C., & Watts, N. (2020). Tracking Infectious Diseases in a Warming World. *BMJ*, *371*, m3086. doi:10.1136/bmj. m3086

Singh, S. K., & Kuhn, J. H. (Eds.) (2019). *Defense Against Biological Attacks: Volume I*. Springer.

Walsh, P. F. (2016). Managing Emerging Health Security Threats Since 9/11: The Role of Intelligence. *International Journal of Intelligence and Counterintelligence*, *29*(2), 341–367.

Walsh, P. F. (2018). *Intelligence, Biosecurity and Bioterrorism*. Springer.

Walsh, P. F. (2020a). Improving 'Five Eyes' Health Security Intelligence Capabilities: Leadership and Governance Challenges. *Intelligence and National Security*, *35*(4), 586–602.

Walsh, P. F. (2020b). *Building a Better Pandemic and Health Security Intelligence Response in Australia*. Centre for International Governance Innovation (August 24th).

Walsh, P. F. (2022). Securing the Bioeconomy: Exploring the Role of Cyberbiosecurity. In Gill, M. (ed.), *The Handbook of Security* (pp. 335–355). Springer International Publishing.

Walsh, P. F., Ramsay, J., & Bernot, A. (2023). Health Security Intelligence Capabilities Post COVID-19: Resisting the Passive "New Normal" Within the Five Eyes. *Intelligence and National Security*, *38*(7), 1095–1111.

Wark, W. (2020). *The System Was Not Blinking Red: Intelligence, Early Warning and Risk Assessment in a Pandemic Crisis*. Centre for International Governance Innovation. www. cigionline.org/articles/system-was-not-blinking-red-intelligence-early-warning-and-risk-assessment-pandemic-crisis/

Wark, W. (2021). Building a Better Global Health Security Early-Warning System Post-COVID: The View from Canada. *International Journal*, *76*(1), 55–67.

West, L., Juneau, T., & Amarasingam, A. (Eds.) (2021). *Stress Tested: The COVID-19 Pandemic and Canadian National Security*. University of Calgary Press.

Wilson, J. M. (2017). Signal Recognition During the Emergence of Pandemic Influenza Type A/H1N1: A Commercial Disease Intelligence Unit's Perspective. *Intelligence and National Security*, *32*(2), 222–230.

Wilson, J. M., Iannarone, M., & Wang, C. (2013). Media Reporting of the Emergence of the 1968 Influenza Pandemic in Hong Kong: Implications for Modern-day Situational Awareness. *Disaster Medicine and Public Health Preparedness*, *3*(S2), S148–S153. doi:10.1097/DMP.0b013e3181abd603

2 Framing National Security and Health Security Intelligence

Erik Dahl

Introduction

Although it might seem surprising, there is little agreement among intelligence professionals about how to define "intelligence," and about what kinds of problems and threats intelligence organizations should concern themselves with. There is also debate over whether medical and public health professionals should be considered to do "intelligence" work, or whether the kinds of disease surveillance and other work they do is similar to, or something quite different from, the work done by traditional national security agencies. This chapter explores and defines these concepts and other key contested terminology, and it provides a foundation for the analysis in later chapters.[1]

The chapter begins by examining the many ways that intelligence professionals and scholars define the term "intelligence," and addresses several fundamental questions about intelligence, such as whether it needs to be secret, and whether it should be considered strictly a function of government. Next, it asks, what are the primary functions of intelligence—what is it used for? Later sections look at how intelligence performs its functions, and whether intelligence can best be thought of as a scientific endeavor, or an artistic one. This is followed by a brief review of the important fields of medical and public health intelligence, and the many similarities between what national security intelligence professionals do and what medical practitioners do. The final sections review the key concepts of intelligence failure and actionable intelligence, and the chapter concludes by drawing lessons from this analysis that can help guide the reader's understanding of the later chapters.

What Is "Intelligence," Anyway?

There are many different ways to define intelligence, and even among intelligence experts there is often little agreement on just what we mean when we talk about "intelligence." Intelligence historian Michael Warner complained a few years ago that "the term is defined anew by each author who addresses it, and these definitions rarely refer to one another or build off what has been written before" (Warner 2002, p. 15). This section examines the debate over how to define intelligence, and poses two key questions: Does intelligence need to be secret? And, is intelligence strictly

DOI: 10.4324/9781003335511-3

a government function, or can it also be carried out by private companies and other organizations?

Defining Intelligence

One aspect that most experts do agree on is that intelligence is different from information. Intelligence is generally considered to be raw data, or information, that has been collected and analyzed for some purpose; or to put it another way, the process of collection and analysis turns raw information into intelligence. And there is also consensus among experts that intelligence can be defined as the sum of its various parts. Mark Lowenthal, for example, writes that intelligence can be thought of as a *process*, by which information is collected and analyzed; as the *product* of that analysis; and as the *organizations* and units that carry out the intelligence function (Lowenthal 2023, 10).

Beyond this, however, there is little agreement about just how to define intelligence. Lowenthal, for example, writes that "intelligence refers to information that meets the stated or understood needs of policy makers and has been collected, processed, and focused to meet those needs" (Lowenthal 2023, 1). This definition is similar to that found in many intelligence textbooks, and at first glance it might seem sufficient. But on a closer look, we can see that Lowenthal's definition is rather narrow—it describes intelligence as something produced specifically to meet the needs of policy makers. This is in line with the idea that intelligence agencies exist primarily to serve senior government leaders; as is often said, the president is "customer number one."[2] But such a definition neglects the use of intelligence to inform consumers beyond the rather rarified audience of government policy makers.

A quite different definition was proposed in 1955 by a task force under a blue-ribbon commission known as the Second Hoover Commission. It stated that "intelligence deals with all the things which should be known in advance of initiating a course of action" (Warner 2002, 16). This broader definition suggests intelligence can encompass much more than decision making by senior government officials. If you want to buy a car, let's say, you gather data from websites, recommendations from friends, or data from other sources—that's raw information—and you make an intelligence assessment about what kind of car would be right for you.

Debates over how to define intelligence are more than just academic arguments. From the point of view of the consumer of intelligence, different definitions of intelligence could put you on very different paths. Do you want your intelligence analysts to be taking a big-picture approach, using all sorts of information to analyze many different kinds of problems? Or do you want your intelligence to be more focused, addressing specific problems and questions that you have identified? And from the point of view of intelligence agencies and professionals, an inability to agree on what we mean by the very term "intelligence" could make it difficult to do the job in a coordinated fashion. As one article put it, without having a common understanding of fundamental concepts, "the intelligence community, quite literally, does not know what it is doing" (Wheaton & Beerbower 2006, 320).

One of the most useful definitions is that proposed by former CIA official Lyman Kirkpatrick, who wrote that intelligence is "the knowledge—and ideally, foreknowledge—sought by nations in response to external threats and to protect their vital interests, especially the well-being of their own people" (Warner 2002, 17). Today, especially in an age when the world is grappling with a wide variety of threats, including health threats, we should broaden that definition to the following: "intelligence is knowledge and foreknowledge sought by a consumer concerning threats to their vital interests." But even this definition, of course, leaves questions to be asked, such as whether or not intelligence must be secret. The next section will begin to address these questions.

Key Questions about Intelligence

One of the most important questions to be asked about intelligence today is: **does it need to be kept secret?** Many experts argue that intelligence fundamentally involves secrets, and that is what makes it distinct. For example, a task force sponsored by the Council on Foreign Relations examined the U.S. intelligence system in 1996, and had this to say:

> Intelligence is information not publicly available, or analysis based at least in part on such information, that has been prepared for policymakers or other actors inside the government. What makes intelligence unique is its use of information that is collected secretly and prepared in a timely manner to meet the needs of policymakers.
>
> (Council on Foreign Relations 1996, 9)

Michael Warner also sees intelligence as fundamentally secret, writing that "without secrets, it is not intelligence" (Warner 2002, 20). This emphasis on secrets is what inspires intelligence agencies to seek to protect "sources and methods," and discourages them from publicizing their work very widely.

But this nearly exclusive focus on secret information has been changing for some time, as intelligence agencies have realized the importance of what is usually called "open-source intelligence." Former CIA deputy director and acting director Michael Morell noted that one of the reasons why the intelligence community failed to anticipate the revolutionary changes in the Middle East that became known as the Arab Spring was that the IC was not paying attention to open-source, unclassified information about unrest growing among Arab populations: "we had become too accustomed to stealing secrets and were not paying enough attention to important information that was streaming on Twitter for the world to see" (Morell 2015, 180).

More recently, the proliferation of unclassified and open-source intelligence, such as commercial satellite imagery, means that, according to two intelligence insiders, "private firms and journalistic outfits now often beat the intelligence community at its own game" (Brown & Medina 2021). And the Russian invasion of Ukraine demonstrated the importance of open source intelligence, as journalists, private companies, and other organizations used a wide variety of sources to track and report on the movements of the Russian military (A New Era of Transparent Warfare 2022). The importance of unclassified, open-source intelligence is even more widely recognized when assessing non-traditional threats and concerns, such as natural disasters and climate change (Briggs, Matejova, & Weiss 2022); and as later chapters of this book will discuss, open-source intelligence is critical in the assessment and tracking of disease threats.

Another question often asked about intelligence is, **who does it?** Traditionally, intelligence has been seen largely as a function of national governments. Warner, for example, concluded following his extensive examination of definitions of intelligence that "intelligence is secret, state activity to understand or influence foreign entities" (Warner 2002, 21). But what then about the role of state and local authorities, or of the private sector?

It remains true that most traditional, national security intelligence work is conducted by nation-states. Intelligence-sharing arrangements are common, such as the 'Five Eyes' partnership involving Australia, Canada, New Zealand, the United Kingdom, and the United States. But still, most fundamental intelligence collection and analysis systems are national. The United Nations, for example, has little intelligence capacity on its own, nor does the North Atlantic Treaty Organization (NATO).

Since the 9/11 terrorist attacks, however, the role of state and local government in intelligence has increased in the U.S. (Dahl 2021b), especially through the growth of a network of 80 state and local intelligence fusion centers, including at least one in every state. The role of private sector intelligence has also greatly increased in recent years (Robson Morrow 2022). As will be discussed in Chapter 10 of this book, the private sector has a particularly important role in providing open-source warning and analysis of disease threats.

What Is Intelligence "For"?

Another question that might seem to have an obvious answer but is actually contested is, what is the purpose of intelligence? What does it do, broadly speaking? Intelligence officials frequently describe their job as "speaking truth to power," and it would seem logical to see the job of intelligence agencies and professionals as that of helping leaders or decisionmakers establish the truth of a situation or problem. This sentiment is captured in a phrase inscribed on the wall of the CIA headquarters building: "And ye shall know the truth, and the truth shall make you free." But even this lofty sentiment is contentious, and Mark Lowenthal has described it as both wrong and dangerous. It is wrong, he writes, because it overstates what intelligence can actually do: "we rarely have a complete picture of a given situation" (Lowenthal 2021, 796). And it is dangerous, because when intelligence professionals misrepresent what they are capable of providing, decision makers may rely on their analysis more than should be warranted, potentially leading to bad policy.

Another popular but problematic view of the role of intelligence is that its job is to predict or forecast the future. This goal is captured in a popular buzzword in

American intelligence: "anticipatory intelligence." But can we expect intelligence agencies to anticipate coming threats and forecast future developments? Former CIA Director John Brennan acknowledged the importance of this role during his Senate confirmation hearings, when he said, "with billions of dollars invested in C.I.A. over the past decade, policymaker expectations of C.I.A.'s ability to antici- pate major geopolitical events should be high" (Mazzetti 2013). But although intelligence experts acknowledge that policy makers will want to know about the future, they are careful to not promise too much. As Harvard professor and former chair of the National Intelligence Council Joseph Nye wrote, "no one can know the future, and it is misleading to pretend to" (Nye 1994, 88).

Another frequently cited goal of intelligence is to understand the enemy. This approach helped contribute to one of the greatest successes in the history of American naval intelligence, before the Battle of Midway in World War II. As the U.S. Navy was attempting to determine where the Japanese fleet was headed, the American commander, Admiral Chester Nimitz, told his senior intelligence officer, LCDR Edwin Layton, that Layton's job was to get inside the mind of the enemy— to "be" the Japanese commander. Layton, who had lived in Japan and was fluent in Japanese, was able to give Nimitz a nearly perfect forecast of how the Japanese would attack Midway, enabling the admiral to position U.S. ships to intercept them.[3] Former Acting CIA Director Michael Morell put it this way:

> An intelligence officer has a lot of different jobs. The main job is to accur- ately describe a situation that a president and his or her national security team, the country faces, to accurately describe that in all of its detail, in all of its complexity. But they also have another job, and the other job is to be able to accurately describe the way the adversary looks at the situation, to be able to tell President Biden, "Here's how President Putin sees the world. Here's how President Putin sees you. Here's how the terrorists see the world. Here's how the terrorists see us."
>
> (Cruickshank 2021, 5)

Intelligence scholar Jennifer Sims takes a similar view, arguing that the purpose of intelligence "is to gain competitive advantage over adversaries—that is, to help one side win over the other" (Sims 2010, 392). Such an approach makes sense when intelligence agencies confront traditional challenges, such as terrorist groups and nation states. But does it apply when the threat comes from a natural disaster, or an infectious disease? There is an "enemy" to be fought, to be sure, but is it appro- priate for intelligence professionals to think about such enemies in the same way?

A broader view sees the job of intelligence to provide a "picture of what is happening in the world," as one of the first heads of the CIA, Hoyt Vandenberg, used to say (Hilsman 1952, 3). Intelligence collects and assembles facts, but importantly, its job is to provide meaning and significance to the facts (Hilsman, 15). And all of this intelligence is intended for a specific purpose: most experts would agree that intelligence exists to assist in planning and decision-making by decision makers. As we have seen, this has traditionally meant senior-level officials, as expressed by

Loch Johnson, who is one of the most respected intelligence scholars in the United States: "put simply, the main purpose of intelligence is to provide information to policymakers that may help illuminate their decision options" (Johnson 2010, 5).

But more often recently, such as concerning health threats including COVID-19, those decision makers have not only been senior government leaders, but they have been local health officials or medical and public health professionals. This broader understanding of who can be considered decision makers was implied in a comment written in the context of the COVID-19 pandemic by David Omand, the former Security and Intelligence Coordinator for the British government and former director of Government Communications Headquarters (GCHQ), the British version of the American National Security Agency (NSA). Omand wrote that "the purpose of having intelligence is to enable better, more timely, decisions by reducing the ignorance of the decision takers" (Omand 2020).

Where Should Intelligence Focus?

Although many governments have used intelligence for internal control—what is often called "security intelligence"—the primary role for national security intelligence in most modern states, including the "Five Eyes" countries, has been to look outside the nation's border at external threats. And although one of the revelations of the Edward Snowden leaks was that American intelligence had evidently listened in on the cell phone of German Chancellor Angela Merkel, it is actually no secret that countries, including allies, do spy on one another.

Although Western democracies have domestic intelligence functions, those roles are typically limited and distinct from the foreign intelligence function. This distinction can be seen in the U.K., for example, in the separate roles assigned to MI-6, which is officially known as the Secret Intelligence Service and serves as the U.K.'s foreign intelligence service; and MI-5, the Security Service, which is a purely domestic intelligence and security agency without any police function. In the United States, most of the agencies of the federal intelligence community are legally limited in what they can collect and do on American soil and on American citizens.

In the first years after the 9/11 attacks, the U.S. national security establishment attempted to maintain a distinction between national security and homeland security, such as by creating a Homeland Security Council, apart from the more traditional National Security Council (NSC). But the Homeland Security Council was within a few years folded back within the NSC, and in recent years this distinction between foreign and domestic has been reduced. But this has raised important legal and ethical dilemmas (examined in Chapter 7), such as how much authority intelligence officials should have in monitoring citizens' social media, and the balance between privacy and security, particularly as it applied in the health security context.

Another important question for intelligence agencies is how much of a focus they should put on nontraditional threats and concerns such as health and infectious disease. Many traditional national security intelligence organizations do indeed collect and analyze information about medical and public health issues. The CIA, for example, has long tracked the health of world leaders and reported on the national security implications of disease outbreaks. And during the COVID-19 pandemic, many Americans learned for the first time of the existence of the U.S. National Center for Medical Intelligence (NCMI), which is a relatively small organization under the Defense Intelligence Agency that provides medical intelligence covering issues ranging from bioterrorist threats to understanding the medical capabilities of countries around the world.

Many intelligence experts argue, however, that traditional intelligence agencies should not be concerned with health issues beyond subjects such as bioterrorism that have a direct nexus to national security. Former senior British intelligence official David Omand has argued that "the assessment of disease outbreaks is not the business of the intelligence community" (Omand 2020). And national security expert Josh Rovner argues that it would be inappropriate and possibly harmful if the IC tried to significantly broaden its focus beyond collecting and analyzing secret information on traditional threats such as from foreign nation-states (Rovner 2021). Such a wider focus, Rovner believes, could duplicate the work done by academics and other analysts and pull scarce resources away from the core threats where intelligence agencies can employ their critical comparative advantage—the ability to provide policy makers with secret information not available anywhere else.

This is related to a debate over the meaning of the term "national security." Should national security include nontraditional threats and concerns such as health and disease? It might seem obvious that national security should indeed include concerns such as health. After all, during the COVID-19 pandemic, many leaders used the language of national security and even war to describe the struggle against it. The United States and many other nations mobilized military forces to combat the virus, and among many other obvious national security effects, the fallout from the pandemic forced an American aircraft carrier to shore in Guam and led to the resignation of the Secretary of the Navy.

But many critics argue that using the language of war and national security to describe a pandemic or other health threat merely securitizes or even militarizes what should instead be treated as a public health problem (Christoyannopoulos 2020). Paul Rogers, for example, has warned about the dangers of "securitizing the pandemic as a threat to be controlled, not a common problem to be addressed cooperatively with an emphasis on aid to the weakest and most marginalized" (Rogers 2020).

Despite these concerns, the Biden administration has clearly signaled that it does consider pandemics to be a matter of national security. It has issued a *National Security Strategy* that calls for greater focus on global public health as well as on preparing for health threats ranging from future pandemics to state-based biological warfare (White House 2022), and called on Congress to provide $88 billion to address the challenges of pandemics and biological threats (Banco 2022). In addition, Congress renamed the National Counter Proliferation Center as the National Counterproliferation and Biosecurity Center, with an expanded mission to include collecting and analyzing intelligence on biological threats (Dilanian 2021).

How Does Intelligence Do Its Job?

This chapter has so far discussed how to define the concept of intelligence, and what it is that intelligence agencies and professionals do. But how do they do their job? How do intelligence analysts learn to understand the world, anticipate threats and challenges, and help leaders and consumers of intelligence make better decisions? The fundamental method used by intelligence is to use a process called the **intelligence cycle**. The cycle begins with intelligence personnel developing a collection plan in response to a requirement or a question from a decision maker; collecting raw information that can help meet that requirement or answer that question; processing and analyzing that information to convert it into an intelligence report or product; and finally, providing that product or other kinds of assessments to decision makers.

Some experts have criticized the intelligence cycle for not representing the way intelligence works in practice. Arthur Hulnick, for example, has written that in the real world, policy makers rarely provide the kind of clear guidance and direction that intelligence analysts are typically taught to expect (Hulnick 2006). And Robert Clark has argued that the model of a cycle appears to make the process seem too linear, with each step occurring one after another, when in actuality everything may be happening at the same time (Clark 2020). But still, the intelligence cycle can be seen like any other model of a system or a process—although it may not provide an exact representation of how that system works, it can be a useful tool in understanding the system. For example, a number of public health authorities have seen the traditional intelligence cycle as a useful way to describe how public health practices can be managed during a health crisis (Bowsher, Bernard, and Sullivan 2020, 440).

Another common method used by intelligence professionals is to attempt to collect indicators, or signals, of potentially dangerous events or actions, in the hopes of being able to provide warning of threats. The job of collecting and analyzing these signals is known as "indications and warning," or I&W, and it is frequently done by military analysts. History has shown that before military forces can conduct significant action, they must make preparations that can be observed by the other side, such as the fueling of aircraft, the assembly of ground troops, or an increase in command and control communications. Before the Russian invasion of Ukraine, for example, U.S. analysts tracked indications of Russian activity (Barnes and Sanger 2022). Such indicators are signs of intent—of what the adversary or competitor is planning to do. Some natural threats put off indicators, such as earthquakes that can to some extent be predicted by the presence of minor shocks ahead of time. But one of the key questions about health security intelligence is whether the collection of indicators and warning can be as effective as it is in other areas of analysis. These questions of whether indicators and warning systems used in more traditional national security threats can be effective in the health security context are discussed further in Chapter 6.

The task of collecting information, sifting through it, and analyzing it for potential threats is often seen as finding signals amidst the noise. In her classic book on

Pearl Harbor Roberta Wohlstetter wrote, "in short, we failed to anticipate Pearl Harbor not for want of the relevant materials, but because of a plethora of irrelevant ones" (Wohlstetter 1962, 387). More recently the 9/11 Commission used a similar phrase when it argued that U.S. intelligence agencies failed to "connect the dots" of all the intelligence held by different parts of the intelligence community in the years and months before the terrorist attacks (National Commission on Terrorist Attacks 2004, 408).

Both of these phrases capture the same concept, that the job of intelligence involves seeking out what is important amid a vast array of confusing and often contradictory information. But we should note that the "connecting the dots" metaphor is resisted by many intelligence insiders, because it appears to suggest that the business of intelligence analysis is little more than child's play. Mark Lowenthal described this phrase as "one of the most unperceptive, misleading, demeaning and mean-spirited things ever said about any intelligence organization" (Lowenthal 2008, 306).

Another important way to describe the work of intelligence is through what are known as the "INTS"—the various disciplines of the intelligence business. These are the collection specialties, through which intelligence agencies collect the raw information that makes up the ingredients of finished intelligence. Some of these specialties are widely recognized, such as human intelligence, or HUMINT, which is the collection of intelligence through contact or communication with individuals themselves. The CIA is the primary HUMINT organization in the United States. Signals intelligence (SIGINT) refers to the collection of a wide variety of kinds of information (signals) transmitted by or to a potential adversary or other subject of collection. SIGINT is so important an intelligence tool that the National Security Agency (NSA), the primary US SIGINT agency, is believed to have the largest budget of any element of the US intelligence community.

Geospatial intelligence, or GEOINT, is the collection of information through imagery or other tools that are able to observe the earth. The primary GEOINT organization in the U.S. intelligence community is the National Geospatial-Intelligence Agency (NGA). A less well-known area of intelligence is measurement and signatures intelligence, or MASINT. This is a highly technical discipline that focuses on the emissions given off by weapons systems, human construction such as factories, or natural and environmental phenomena. There is no separate MASINT agency in the U.S. intelligence system. Finally, as has been mentioned earlier in this chapter, another key intelligence source is known as open-source intelligence (OSINT). Although intelligence agencies have long collected information from open and unclassified sources, OSINT has traditionally been seen as secondary to—and not quite as respectable as—classified sources. OSINT collection is coordinated within the U.S. intelligence community by an organization within the CIA called the Open Source Enterprise. But because OSINT is growing in importance, some experts argue that it deserves to be given its own agency. Intelligence expert Amy Zegart and former CIA Acting Director Michael Morell write, "open-source intelligence will never get the focus and funding it requires as long as it sits inside the CIA or any other existing agency" (Zegart and Morell 2019, 95).

An important distinction is often made between **strategic and tactical intelligence**. Strategic intelligence tends to look at longer-term, broader issues, while tactical intelligence addresses narrower focused and typically shorter-term problems. Many experts and leaders say they prefer strategic intelligence, but it is not clear that such warning is actually as effective as tactical intelligence and tactical warning. In the context of health security, strategic intelligence often assesses the danger from potential future outbreaks and pandemics, while tactical intelligence warns about a specific virus or other disease threat that is developing.

One additional concept is important in understanding the role and functioning of intelligence: the relationship between **intelligence and policy**. There is a large literature examining the factors that can make intelligence more effective in gaining the attention of policy makers and other consumers of intelligence. The political scientist Robert Jervis suggests that timing can be critical: "for intelligence to be welcomed and to have an impact, it must arrive at the right time, which is after leaders have become seized with the problem but before they have made up their minds" (Jervis 2010, 196). Studies of the COVID-19 pandemic have found that a strong intelligence-policy relationship appears to have been one factor that contributed to quick, effective action among countries including South Korea, Taiwan, Vietnam, and Germany (Dahl 2023, 104).

But this relationship is seen as something of a paradox. On the one hand, intelligence is widely seen as being of no value if it does not get to someone who can make use of it; in other words, there needs to be a close relationship between intelligence professionals and leaders and other consumers of the intelligence they produce. On the other hand, a too close relationship can be counter-productive, because it could cause the analyst to lose his or her objectivity. Analytic objectivity is seen as necessary for analysts to be able to provide decision makers with unbiased, accurate intelligence. In addition, objectivity is required because intelligence personnel are expected to remain out of policy debates. Mark Lowenthal expresses the relationship between intelligence and policy this way: "in the ethos of U.S. intelligence, a strict dividing line exists between intelligence and policy… . Intelligence has a support role and may not cross over into the advocacy of policy choices" (Lowenthal 2023, 4).

There is a debate among intelligence experts over just how close the relationship should be between intelligence professionals and the policy makers they serve, but in general it is seen as important to keep some distance. Sherman Kent, widely considered to be the father of intelligence analysis, and for whom the CIA's Sherman Kent School for Intelligence Analysis is named, believed that there needed to be a strict separation between intelligence and policy (Davis 2002). Kent wrote "intelligence must be close enough to policy, plans, and operations to have the greatest amount of guidance, and must not be so close that it loses its objectivity and integrity of judgement" (Dahl 2021a, 176).

Is Intelligence an Art, or a Science?

Beginning during the Cold War and continuing until today, there has been an effort by intelligence experts and scholars to put intelligence on a scientific footing, and in particular to treat the job of intelligence analysis as a social science (National Research Council 2011).

But there are other experts who believe that intelligence is as much an art as it is a science, and that it would be a mistake to try to make it too scientific. *New York Times* columnist David Brooks, for example, has argued that the intelligence community tries too hard to be scientific and quantitative, which is not the right way to analyze and understand human behavior (Brooks 2005), while former Pentagon official Elbridge Colby has criticized the CIA's "deep ardor for political science" (Colby 2007).

One view is that the work of intelligence focuses primarily on human-caused threats and dangers, while much of science is concerned with natural hazards and challenges. Similarly, some experts make a distinction between **threats** as referring to human-caused dangers, and **hazards**, which are naturally caused. A RAND study described the concepts this way: "*threats* are defined as events that result from an individual or group with both the intent and capability to cause harm. Threats include terrorism and illegal activities. In contrast to threats, *hazards* refers to naturally occurring events that lead to harm" (Willis et al. 2018, 3–4).

Despite these distinctions, the U.S. intelligence community has for many years worked closely with scientists and scientific groups. One area of coordination has been in the area of climate science and environmental research; in 1992 intelligence agencies worked with climate scientists in what was called the Environmental Task Force, and in 1994 the ETF evolved into a scientific advisory group known as MEDEA (Barnard, Johnson, and Porter 2021). And more recently the National Academies of Sciences, Engineering, and Medicine established a Climate Security Roundtable, to bring together scientists and the IC to study ways climate change affects U.S. national security.[4]

Today, however, intelligence agencies are turning to scientists more often, as they are asked about issues and topics that have not normally been high on their agenda (Barnes 2021b). Examples include studies about Unidentified Flying Objects (Williams, Cohen, and Herb 2021), and about health issues including the cause of the mysterious Havana Syndrome attacks (Vergano 2021), and about the origins of the COVID-19 pandemic (Barnes 2021a). The connections between intelligence and the scientific community and how they might be fostered further is discussed in Chapter 8.

Medical and Public Health Intelligence

Thus far, this chapter has focused on traditional national security intelligence concepts and organizations, which as we have seen often deal with threats related to health and disease. But as later chapters will discuss in more detail, health problems such as pandemics are primarily addressed by medical and public health organizations and systems that are not formally linked to the national security intelligence community.

There is a long history of intelligence and surveillance in medicine and public health, and in fact surveillance is seen as a key part of public health. Former CDC director David Satcher writes, "in public health, we can't do anything without sur-veillance. That's where public health begins" (Centers for Disease Control and Prevention nd, 35). Public health surveillance typically means the systematic collection and analysis on data concerning infectious diseases, but it can also be used to track other health issues, including chronic diseases.

The language used to describe public health surveillance is often similar to that used for national security intelligence. For example, Henry Rolka and Kara Contreary write, "the purpose of public health surveillance is to support sound decision making in order to prevent or control the spread of disease in a popula-tion" (Rolka and Contreary 2016, 22; see also Bowsher, Milner, Sullivan 2016). A number of experts in national security intelligence have noted a similarity between what they do and what medical practitioners do. Stephen Marrin and Jonathan D. Clemente, for example, have examined lessons from the medical profession that can be used for improving intelligence analysis (Marrin and Clemente 2005). There has been less research done from the opposite perspec-tive, but nonetheless some medical experts have described what they do in terms of intelligence. Others have used the intelligence cycle to describe the functions of public health (Bowsher, Bernard, and Sullivan 2020). Still, some medical and public health practitioners resist being labelled as part of an intelligence effort, and as we have seen above, critics of the "securitization" of medicine and public health argue it is wrong to see pandemics through a wartime lens (Nordstom and Senk 2022).

Despite the differences between national security and health security intelli-gence, professionals in both fields are often criticized for failing to use the tools at their disposal to anticipate and prevent threats from arising. The next section examines the concept of intelligence failure, and how it has been applied to both national and health security intelligence.

What Is Intelligence Failure?

The topic of intelligence failure is one of the most widely discussed in the study of intelligence, and it is something of a sore subject for many intelligence professionals. Former U.S. Marine Corps intelligence director Lieutenant General Paul van Riper complained that "the Intelligence Community does a damn good job. It troubles me that people always speak in terms of operational successes and intelligence failures" (Dahl 2013, 6). This view is not surprising, because intelli-gence failures are more widely publicized than intelligence successes, since pub-licizing successes may expose sources and methods that are still being used. As President John F. Kennedy said in a speech to CIA employees, "your successes are unheralded—your failures are trumpeted" (Kennedy 1961).

Intelligence failure is another contested term, with little agreement among intel-ligence professionals or national security experts on just what should be considered an intelligence failure. The classic case for national security intelligence is the failure to warn about or prevent a surprise attack, such as Pearl Harbor or 9/11. In the health security intelligence context, an example of failure was the intelligence community's inability to understand the size, scope, and sophistication of the Soviet Union's biological weapons (BW) program during the Cold War. This failure only came to light following the defection to the West of senior Soviet BW officials, including Ken Alibek, in the late 1980s and early 1990s (Koblentz 2009, 157–169). Happily, for the West, the uncomfortable surprise revelation of the full nature of the Soviet BW program did not result in disaster, but the episode was an example of the challenges for intelligence in assessing health security threats.

Major recent intelligence failures include the inability to properly assess Iraq's weapons of mass destruction program in 2003, to anticipate the spread of pro-democracy movements in the Middle East that became the Arab Spring, and to understand the rise of ISIS in 2013 and 2014. Mark Lowenthal defines the term this way: "an intelligence failure is the inability of one or more parts of the intelligence process—collection, evaluation and analysis, production, dissemination—to produce timely, accurate intelligence on an issue or event of importance to national interests." (Lowenthal 1985, 51).

But this definition begs the question: is it enough for intelligence simply to have warned of a threat? This was the argument made by Capitol Police intelligence official Julie Farnam, who said after the January 6 attack on the Capitol, "I think we provided the information. I think we did an excellent job" (Kaplan and Van Cleave 2022). The problem is that after terrorist attacks, mass shootings, and other disasters, we almost always learn that there had been warnings in the pipeline. This is what James Wirtz has termed the "first law of intelligence failure"—that there is almost always found to have been some warning before bad things happen (Wirtz 2006, 51). The question is, where should we set the goalposts; how much warning is enough?

Before the COVID-19 pandemic, a number of intelligence leaders and other experts warned about the threat of a global pandemic. The U.S. National Intelligence Council, for example, published in 2008 a remarkably prescient scenario about how in 2025 a pandemic starting in Asia could produce millions of deaths in the United States alone (Dahl 2023, 88). And more recently, then-Director of National Intelligence Dan Coats testified in 2019 that "the world will remain vulnerable to the next flu pandemic or large-scale outbreak of a contagious disease that could lead to massive rates of death and disability (Coats 2019, 21). Is such warning enough to mean there was no intelligence failure? This argument has been made by a number of intelligence experts. Calder Walton, for example, has written that the pandemic was not an intelligence failure, because intelligence agencies had been warning (Walton 2020). And according to James Wirtz, "it is clear that COVID-19 cannot be characterized as an intelligence failure, or as a failure of public health officials or the security studies community to understand the general course and consequences of the threat. The possibility of a global pandemic was not only predictable, it was also predicted by the scientific (and intelligence) community" (Wirtz 2021, 129).

But other experts from the fields of intelligence, medicine, and public health have argued that the pandemic did represent a failure of intelligence, because even though many agencies and analysts saw a pandemic coming, their warnings either failed to be heard, or had little impact on those who did listen to them (Levy and Wark, 2021; O'Toole and Bourdeaux, 2020). This view relies on definition of intelligence failure that I have offered in previous work (Dahl 2013, 7), which sees intelligence failure as involving either a failure of intelligence to provide intelligence needed by decision makers, or a failure by decision makers to act on that intelligence appropriately. Seen that way, the COVID-19 pandemic can be considered as an intelligence failure.

However one defines intelligence failure, the goal for intelligence producers and consumers alike is clearly to avoid failure. How can we do better next time? Part of the answer may be found in another concept familiar to national security intelligence professionals: actionable intelligence.

Actionable Intelligence

One of the most popular buzzwords in recent years has been actionable intelligence. It is highly sought after, and intelligence failures are often equated with a lack of actionable intelligence. For example, President George W. Bush told the 9/11 Commission in a 2004 interview that prior to the 9/11 attacks "there was no actionable intelligence on such a threat—not one" (Volz and Strobel 2022). In addition, the Department of Homeland Security Inspector General found that before the January 6, 2021, assault on the Capitol, DHS was unable to provide actionable intelligence (Department of Homeland Security Office of the Inspector General 2022). The lack of actionable intelligence has also been seen in the context of health problems; two medical and public health experts wrote after the Ebola crisis of 2014 that "the common thread underlying failures associated with such public health crises is deficiencies in actionable intelligence that inform process, policy, and responsiveness" (Carney and Weber 2015, 1740).

The link between intelligence and action seems clear. As British intelligence expert R. V. Jones has written, "the ultimate object of Intelligence is to enable action to be optimized" (Jones 1989, 288). But what is actionable intelligence? It too is a contested term. One expert defines it as intelligence that "is highly valued as being timely and detailed enough to give decision-makers a decision advantage in being able to act quickly" (George 2020, 295). Sometimes the term seems to be used as a shorthand to describe any intelligence that is valuable or desirable. The Department of Defense *Dictionary of Military and Associated Terms,* for example, defines actionable intelligence as: "intelligence information that is directly useful to customers for immediate exploitation without having to go through the full intelligence production process" (Department of Defense 2016, 1).

Two key factors appear to be necessary in order for intelligence to be actionable. First, actionable intelligence is specific intelligence—what in a military and national security context would be called tactical intelligence. And second, it needs to satisfy a need or requirement for a decision maker. Perhaps the most useful definition comes from Loch Johnson, who writes that actionable intelligence is "specific enough to allow policy officials to act upon the information" (Johnson 2010, 21).

Conclusion

Much of the rest of this book can be seen as an effort to determine how the world can provide better, more actionable intelligence and warning for the next global pandemic or other major health security threats, risks and hazards. But the analysis of this chapter can offer us several provisional conclusions.

First, actionable intelligence in the area of health security must be broad-based, not relying solely on classified national security intelligence. It must be the product of an all-source and whole of society effort including sources from epidemiology, public health surveillance, and scientific research conducted by government as well as private sector experts.

Second, in order for intelligence to be truly actionable—to be able to help policy makers make decisions, and to help provide for health security and prevent crises such as pandemics from happening—it must provide specific, tactical-level warning, and it must be received by decision makers who have enough trust in and understanding of their intelligence professionals that they are able to make an educated decision.

Notes

1 Some portions of this chapter are drawn from my recent work (Dahl, 2023).
2 For example, this is how then-Director of National Intelligence James Clapper described the president in 2016 (Clapper 2016).
3 This story has been often told, such as in (Dahl, 2013, pp. 60–61).
4 See for example, https://www.nationalacademies.org/our-work/climate-security-roundtable.

References

A New Era of Transparent Warfare (2022). A New Era of Transparent Warfare Beckons: Russia's Manoeuvres are a Coming-Out Party for Open-Source Intelligence. *Economist*. www.economist.com/briefing/2022/02/18/a-new-era-of-transparent-warfare-beckons

Banco, E. (2022). Biden Admin Unveils New Pandemic Preparedness and Biodefense Strategy. *Politico*. www.politico.com/news/2022/10/18/biden-pandemic-biodefense-strategy-00062207

Barnard, E., Johnson, L. K., & Porter, J. (2021). Environmental Security Intelligence: The Role of US Intelligence Agencies and Science Advisory Groups in Anticipating Climate Security Threats. *Journal of Intelligence History*. https://doi.org/10.1080/16161262.2021.2021687

Barnes, J. E. (2021a). Origin of Virus May Remain Murky, U.S. Intelligence Agencies Say. *New York Times*. www.nytimes.com/2021/10/29/us/politics/coronavirus-origin-intelligence-report.html

Barnes, J. E. (2021b). Spy Agencies Turn to Scientists as They Wrestle with Mysteries. *New York Times*. www.nytimes.com/2021/07/08/us/politics/intelligence-agencies-science.html?action=click&module=Spotlight&pgtype=Homepage

Barnes, J. E., & Sanger, D. E. (2022). Accurate U.S. intelligence Did Not Stop Putin, But it Gave Biden Big Advantages. *New York Times*. www.nytimes.com/2022/02/24/world/europe/intelligence-putin-biden-ukraine-leverage.html

Betts, R. K. (1978). Analysis, War, and Decision: Why Intelligence Failures are Inevitable. *World Politics*, *31*(1), 61–89.

Bowsher, G., Bernard, R., & Sullivan, R. (2020). A Health Intelligence Framework for Pandemic Response: Lessons From the UK Experience of COVID-19. *Health Security*, *18*(6), 435–443. https://doi.org/10.1089/hs.2020.0108

Bowsher, G., Milner, C., & Sullivan, R. (2016). Medical Intelligence, Security and Global Health: The Foundations of a New Health Agenda. *Journal of the Royal Society of Medicine*, *109*(7), 269–273.

Briggs, C. M., Matejova, M., & Weiss, R. (2022). Disaster Intelligence: Developing Strategic Warning for National Security. *Intelligence and National Security*. https://doi.org/10.1080/02684527.2022.2043080

Brooks, D. (2005). The Art of Intelligence. *New York Times*. www.nytimes.com/2005/04/02/opinion/the-art-of-intelligence.html

Brown, Z. T., & Medina, C. A. (2021). The Declining Market for Secrets: U.S. Spy Agencies Must Adapt to an Open-Source World. *Foreign Affairs*. www.foreignaffairs.com/articles/united-states/2021-03-09/declining-market-secrets

Carney, T. J., & Weber, D. J. (2015). Public Health Intelligence: Learning from the Ebola Crisis. *American Journal of Public Health*, *105*(9), 1740–1744.

Centers for Disease Control and Prevention (n.d.). *Public Health Surveillance: Preparing for the Future*. www.cdc.gov/surveillance/pdfs/Surveillance-Series-Bookleth.pdf

Christoyannopoulos, A. (2020). Stop Calling Coronavirus Pandemic a "War." *The Conversation*. https://theconversation.com/stop-calling-coronavirus-pandemic-a-war-135486

Clapper, J. R. (2016). *U.S. Intelligence as a Pillar of Stability During Transition*. INSA and AFCEA Intelligence & National Security Summit. www.dni.gov/index.php/newsroom/speeches-interviews/speeches-interviews-2016/item/1627-dni-clapper-s-as-delivered-remarks-at-the-2016-insa-afcea-intelligence-national-security-summit

Clark, R. M. (2020). *Intelligence Analysis: A Target-Centric Approach*. CQ Press.

Coats, D. R. (2019). Worldwide Threat Assessment of the US Intelligence Community. (Senate Select Committee on Intelligence, January 29). www.dni.gov/files/ODNI/documents/2019-ATA-SFR---SSCI.pdf

Colby, E. A. (2007). *Making Intelligence Smart*. Hoover Institution. www.hoover.org/research/making-intelligence-smart

Copeland, T. E. (2017). Intelligence Failure Theory. *Oxford Research Encyclopedia of International Studies*. http://oxfordre.com/internationalstudies/view/10.1093/acrefore/9780190846626.001.0001/acrefore-9780190846626-e-27

Council on Foreign Relations (1996). *Making Intelligence Smarter* (Report of an Independent Task Force). Council on Foreign Relations. www.cfr.org/report/making-intelligence-smarter

Cruickshank, P., Rassler, D., & Hummel, K. (2021). Twenty Years After 9/11: Reflections from Michael Morell, Former Acting Director of the CIA. *CTC Sentinel*, *14*(7), 1–5.

Dahl, E. J. (2013). *Intelligence and Surprise Attack: Failure and Success from Pearl Harbor to 9/11 and Beyond*. Georgetown University Press.

Dahl, E. J. (2018). Not Your Father's Intelligence Failure: Why the Intelligence Community Failed to Anticipate the Rise of ISIS. In F. al-Istrabadi & S. Ganguly (Eds.), *The Future of ISIS: Regional and International Implications* (pp. 41–65). Brookings Institution Press.

Dahl, E. J. (2021a). Intelligence and the Theory of Preventive Action. In J. D. Ramsay, K. Cozine, & J. Comiskey (Eds.), *Theoretical Foundations of Homeland Security: Strategies, Operations, and Structures* (pp. 168–186). Routledge.

Dahl, E. J. (2021b). The Localization of Intelligence: A New Direction for American Federalism. *International Journal of Intelligence and Counterintelligence, 34*(1), 151–178. https://doi.org/10.1080/08850607.2020.1716563

Dahl, E. J. (2022). Lessons Learned From the January 6th Intelligence Failures. *Just Security.* www.justsecurity.org/83245/lessons-learned-from-the-january-6th-intelligence-failures/

Dahl, E. J. (2023). *The COVID-19 Intelligence Failure: Why Warning Was Not Enough.* Georgetown University Press.

Davis, J. (2002). *Sherman Kent and the Profession of Intelligence Analysis* (Vol. 1, Number 5; Occasional Papers). Sherman Kent Center for Intelligence Analysis. www.cia.gov/resources/csi/static/Kent-Profession-Intel-Analysis.pdf

Department of Defense (2016). *Department of Defense Dictionary of Military and Associated Terms* (Joint Publication JP 1–02).

Department of Homeland Security Office of the Inspector General (2022). *I&A Identified Threats Prior to January 6, 2021, but Did Not Issue Any Intelligence Products Before the U.S. Capitol Breach (REDACTED)* (OIG-22–29). www.oig.dhs.gov/sites/default/files/assets/2022-04/OIG-22-29-Mar22-Redacted.pdf

Dilanian, K. (2021). House Votes to Create Office for Medical Intelligence to Get Earlier Pandemic Warnings. *NBC News.* www.nbcnews.com/politics/national-security/house-votes-create-new-office-medical-intelligence-get-earlier-pandemic-n1280498

George, R. Z. (2020). *Intelligence in the National Security Enterprise: An Introduction.* Georgetown University Press.

Hilsman, R. (1952). Intelligence and Policy-Making in Foreign Affairs. *World Politics, 5*(1), 1–45. https://doi.org/10.2307/2009086

Hulnick, A. S. (2006). What's Wrong with the Intelligence Cycle. *Intelligence and National Security, 21*(6), 959–979. https://doi.org/10.1080/02684520601046291

Jervis, R. (2010). *Why Intelligence Fails: Lessons from the Iranian Revolution and the Iraq War.* Cornell University Press.

Johnson, L. K. (2010). National Security Intelligence. In L. K. Johnson (Ed.), *The Oxford Handbook of National Security Intelligence* (pp. 3–32). Oxford University Press. https://doi.org/10.1093/oxfordhb/9780195375886.003.0001

Jones, R. V. (1989). Intelligence and Command. In M. I. Handel (Ed.), *Leaders and Intelligence* (pp. 288–298). Routledge.

Kaplan, M., & Van Cleave, K. (2022). Capitol Police Intelligence Official Says She Sounded Alarm About Potential Violence Days Before January 6 Riot. *CBS News.* www.cbsnews.com/news/capitol-police-intelligence-official-julie-farnam-january-6-riot/

Kennedy, J. F. (1961). *Remarks Upon Presenting as Award to Allen W. Dulles.* www.presidency.ucsb.edu/documents/remarks-upon-presenting-award-allen-w-dulles

Koblentz, G. D. (2009). *Living Weapons: Biological Warfare and International Security.* Cornell University Press.

Levy, A. R., & Wark, W. (2021). *The Pandemic Caught Canada Unawares: It Was an Intelligence Failure.* Centre for International Governance Innovation. www.cigionline.org/articles/the-pandemic-caught-canada-unawares-it-was-an-intelligence-failure/

Lowenthal, M. M. (1985). The Burdensome Concept of Failure. In A. C. Maurer, M. D. Tunstall, & James. M. Keagle (Eds.), *Intelligence: Policy and Process* (p. 43–56). Westview Press.

Lowenthal, M. M. (2008). Towards a Reasonable Standard for Analysis: How Right, How Often on Which Issues? *Intelligence and National Security, 23*(3), 303–315. https://doi.org/10.1080/02684520802121190

Lowenthal, M. M. (2021). Intelligence is NOT About "Telling Truth to Power." *International Journal of Intelligence and Counter Intelligence, 34*(4), 795–798. https://doi.org/10.1080/08850607.2021.1928438

Lowenthal, M. M. (2023). *Intelligence: From Secrets to Policy* (9th ed.). CQ Press.

Marrin, S., & Clemente, J. D. (2005). Improving Intelligence Analysis by Looking to the Medical Profession. *International Journal of Intelligence and Counter Intelligence, 18*(4), 707–729. https://doi.org/10.1080/08850600590945434

Mazzetti, M. (2013). New Terror Strategy Shifts C.I.A. Focus Back to Spying. *New York Times.* www.nytimes.com/2013/05/24/us/politics/plan-would-orient-cia-back-toward-spying.html

Morell, M. (2015). *The Great War of Our Time.* Twelve.

National Commission on Terrorist Attacks (2004). *The 9/11 Commission Report.* WW Norton.

National Research Council (2011). *Intelligence Analysis for Tomorrow: Advances from the Behavioral and Social Sciences.* National Academies Press.

Nordstrom, L., & Senk, S. (2022). The Trouble with Viewing 9/11 and the Pandemic Through a Wartime Lens. *Washington Post.* www.washingtonpost.com/outlook/2022/09/09/covid-911-anniversary-war-metaphors/

Nye, J. S. (1994). Peering into the Future. *Foreign Affairs, 73*(4), 82–93. https://doi.org/10.2307/20046745

Omand, D. (2020). Will the Intelligence Agencies Spot the Next Outbreak? *The Article.* www.thearticle.com/will-the-intelligence-agencies-spot-the-next-outbreak

O'Toole, T., & Bourdeaux, M. (2020). *Intelligence Failure? How Divisions Between Intelligence and Public Health Left Us Vulnerable to a Pandemic* (Webinar). Belfer Center. www.belfercenter.org/event/intelligence-failure-how-divisions-between-intellige nce-and-public-health-left-us-vulnerable

Ramsay, J. D., Cozine, K., & Comiskey, J. (Eds.) (2020). *Theoretical Foundations of Homeland Security: Strategies, Operations, and Structures* (1st ed.). Routledge.

Robson Morrow, M. A. (2022). Private Sector Intelligence: On the Long Path of Professionalization. *Intelligence and National Security, 37*(3), 402–420. https://doi.org/10.1080/02684527.2022.2029099

Rogers, P. (2020). COVID-19: The Dangers of Securitisation. *Oxford Research Group (Blog).* /www.oxfordresearchgroup.org.uk/covid-19-the-dangers-of-securitisation

Rolka, H., & Contreary, K. (2016). Past Contributions. In S. J. McNabb, J. M. Conde, L. Ferland, W. MacWright, Z. A. Memish, S. Okutani, M. M. Park, P. Ryland, A. T. Shaikh, & V. Singh (Eds.), *Transforming Public Health Surveillance: Proactive Measures for Prevention, Detection, and Response.* Elsevier.

Rovner, J. (2021). Think Small: Why the Intelligence Community Should Do Less About New Threats. *War on the Rocks.* https://warontherocks.com/2021/06/think-small-why-the-intelligence-community-should-do-less-about-new-threats/

Sims, J. E. (2010). Decision Advantage and the Nature of Intelligence Analysis. In L. K. Johnson (Ed.), *The Oxford Handbook of National Security Intelligence* (pp. 389–403). Oxford University Press. https://doi.org/10.1093/oxfordhb/9780195375886.003.0024

The White House (2022). *National Security Strategy.* www.whitehouse.gov/wp-cont ent/uploads/2022/10/Biden-Harris-Administrations-National-Security-Strategy-10.2022.pdf

Vergano, D. (2021). A Declassified State Department Report Says Microwaves Didn't Cause "Havana Syndrome." *BuzzFeed News.* www.buzzfeednews.com/article/danvergano/hav ana-syndrome-jason-crickets

Volz, D., & Strobel, W. P. (2022). U.S. Releases 9/11 Commission Interview with George W. Bush, Dick Cheney. *Wall Street Journal*. www.wsj.com/articles/u-s-expected-to-rele ase-9-11-commission-interview-with-bush-and-cheney-11668018211

Walton, C. (2020). *US Intelligence, the Coronavirus and the Age of Globalized Challenges*. Centre for International Governance Innovation. www.cigionline.org/articles/us-intellige nce-coronavirus-and-age-globalized-challenges

Warner, M. (2002). Wanted: A definition of 'Intelligence'. *Studies in Intelligence*, *46*(3), 15–22.

Wheaton, K. J., & Beerbower, M. T. (2006). Towards a New Definition of Intelligence. *Stanford Law & Policy Review*, 17(2), 319–330.

Williams, K. B., Cohen, Z., & Herb, J. (2021). US Intelligence Community Releases Long-Awaited UFO Report. *CNN*. www.cnn.com/2021/06/25/politics/ufo-report-pentagon-odni

Willis, H. H., Tighe, M., Lauland, A., Ecola, L., Shelton, S. R., Smith, M. L., Rivers, J. G., Leuschner, K. J., Marsh, T., & Gerstein, D. M. (2018). *Homeland Security National Risk Characterization: Risk Assessment Methodology*. RAND Corporation. www.rand.org/pubs/research_reports/RR2140.html

Wirtz, J. J. (2006). Responding to surprise. *Annual Review of Political Science*, *9*, 45–65.

Wirtz, J. J. (2021). COVID-19: Observations for contemporary strategists. *Defence Studies*, *21*(2), 127–140. https://doi.org/10.1080/14702436.2021.1896361

Wohlstetter, R. (1962). *Pearl Harbor: Warning and Decision*. Stanford University Press.

Zegart, A., & Morell, M. (2019). Spies, Lies, and Algorithms: Why U.S. Intelligence Must Adapt or Fail. *Foreign Affairs*, *98*(3), 85–96.

Part II

Challenges in Managing Health Security Threats, Risks and Hazards

3 Political Engagement

Patrick F. Walsh and Ausma Bernot

Introduction

This chapter surveys the political and institutional barriers that have constrained 'Five Eyes' intelligence agencies in playing consistent and effective roles in managing health security threats and risks, from 9/11 up to and including COVID-19. Building on the fundamental principles discussed in Erik Dahl's chapter (Chapter 2), we demonstrate that the lack of sustained political attention and coordinated policy action on health security issues since 9/11 has left each of the 'Five Eyes' countries, to varying degrees, unprepared to deal with the significant impact of COVID 19. We argue that in most cases this absence of a consistent strategic and operational approach to health security risks, threats and hazards—particularly at the political level—resulted in an equally deficient investment in capabilities within 'Five Eyes' intelligence communities. Such shortcomings, as well as the lack of robust centrally coordinated collection and analytical structures on health security intelligence within Five Eyes ICs, limited their ability to fully participate in supporting whole-of-government efforts (including those led by public health agencies) to warn, prepare, mitigate, and manage the impact of COVID-19. The discussion here lays the foundation for Chapter 5 (Bowsher), which outlines how 'Five Eyes' intelligence agencies might begin to address these political and institutional barriers post-COVID-19.

Political Engagement and Policy Action

Before assessing the political engagement, institutional and policy action challenges, it is important to contextualise how the terms 'health security' and 'health security intelligence' have been used since 9/11. As discussed in Dahl's chapter the notion of what is and isn't 'health security' remains contested. From a contextual perspective, since the 1990s, human security scholars have perceived disease outbreaks in security terms due to their impacts not only on health systems but also their potential to destabilize national economies and disrupt social life (Human Security Centre 2006). We argue that 'health security' is an overarching term that may be used to examine the security implications of both the security and public health aspects of health incidents. Not all health security situations will

DOI: 10.4324/9781003335511-5

involve the same mix of public health, intelligence, and security personnel; nonetheless, however, both dimensions are intertwined (Walsh 2020). Health security intelligence refers to the collection of health security information, utilized before and during the occurrence of the incidents. Health security intelligence prioritizes three types of biosecurity threats—rapidly spreading infectious diseases, bioterrorism, and the potential weaponizing of dual use laboratory research (Walsh 2020). Health security threats are complex issues that require a multi-stakeholder model of work between public health, national security, and intelligence communities to better facilitate and manage emergency warnings and responses. There have been examples of such collaborations between the national security intelligence, public health and scientific communities with the most well-known publicly being the FBI collaboration with the CDC during the 'Amerithrax' (Anthrax investigation), which lasted over seven years (The US Department of Justice 2010). However as will be discussed shortly, such collaborations during the period from 9/11 up to and including COVID-19 have not been consistent or optimal in their effectiveness.

The Amerithrax investigation nonetheless established new pathways for IC agencies, public and other scientific personnel to collaborate more effectively with 29 government, university, and commercial labs augmenting the FBI effort to 'develop the physical, chemical, genetic and forensic profiles of anthrax spores, letters and envelopes used in the attack' (The US Department of Justice 2010, 5). However, it also exposed difficulties between multi-stakeholder government agencies in working effectively together. For example, the FBI tasked geneticist Paul Keim to identify the Anthrax strain used by the attacker. Keim, in a subsequent interview, discussed the challenges in converting his academic lab into a forensic one, and some of the difficulties with the scientific and investigative communities working together including the natural desire of scientists to share knowledge between peers vs. the security needs of the investigation to restrict information flows. Additional challenges included handling scientific material in a way that preserved the evidence from a law enforcement perspective, different from routine scientific protocols (Bhattacharjee 2009, 1416). We argue that, while operational challenges are to be expected during a multi-disciplinary investigation, they are symptomatic of broader, longer-term political/policy and institutional barriers that have periodically inhibited IC responses to biothreats since the immediate aftermath of 9/11, when Amerithrax occurred, and before COVID-19.

The first section of the chapter will survey briefly the key political/policy barriers to consistent and effective IC responses to health security threats and risks from 9/11 up to COVID-19. The focus is almost exclusively on the US and the UK for two reasons. First, space is limited and providing exhaustive coverage of all 'Five Eyes' political and policy activities would not be possible in one chapter. Second, a more significant amount of information is available publicly from the UK and US as successive governments implemented various political and policy initiatives to better manage health security threats and risks.

The second section of the chapter section builds on the analysis by thematically exploring how key policy initiatives may have influenced the ICs' ability to play a consistent and coherent role in supporting the management of health security threats and risks from 9/11 up to COVID-19. We cannot fully know the specific impact of all key policy initiatives on the ICs of the UK and US given much of the details are sensitive or classified. However, there is sufficient publicly available evidence to thematically identify how various factors constrained ICs' ability to play a consistently effective role in the national health security strategy. In the forthcoming section, we turn our attention to an analysis of key political and policy initiatives from 9/11 up to COVID-19 for the UK and US respectively.

9/11 to COVID-19: The United Kingdom and the United States Health Security Policy and Practice

United Kingdom Political and Policy Initiatives

The UK government's historic interest in health security threats and risks extends back to the 1930s with concerns that state actors would use a biological bomb in warfare. There were growing concerns that Nazi Germany was developing a bioweapons program. This resulted in policy attention that would support the development of both defensive and offensive bioweapons at Porton Down (Wiltshire) during 1940–45 (Balmer 2002). This research was carried out in closer collaboration with other 'Five Eyes' partners namely the United States and Canada that were developing similar programs (Carus 2017; Regis 1999; Spiers 2010). However, policy-making priorities soon shifted after World War Two to a mainly defensive program from 1955–1960. As the Cold War brought in a key concern in London and other 'Five Eyes' capitals over the Soviet Union's expanding nuclear weapons capacity, interest in biowarfare began to diminish on the policy agenda (Carus 2017; Regis 1999; Spiers 2010).

From this narrow military view of health security threats and risks, i.e. bioweapons used in conventional warfare, in the period leading up to 9/11 successive UK governments gradually expanded their interpretation and attention towards a broader set of health security threats and risks. These reflected a domestic and international concern over infectious diseases, biosecurity, and bioterrorism. In particular, both the 9/11 attacks and the Amerithrax incident in the US served as catalysts for greater political and policy engagement by UK governments in assessing the intent and capability of non-state actor terrorist groups such as Al Qaeda to use bioweapons. Alongside, there was a growing concern that rogue states like Saddam Hussein's Iraq may possess bioweapons, even though the UN weapons inspection team failed to locate them after the Gulf War in 1991.

The growing concern about bioterrorism was in part the reason for the UK government establishing the Health Protection Agency (HPA) in 2004 (Nicoll & Murray 2002, 129–130). Its role was to bring better coordination between national and regional public levels as well as harness the expertise of other 'non-health' groups and stakeholders essential to health protection (Nicoll & Murray 2002, 131). During this early post-9/11 period, the HPA represented the only major institutional change to create greater coordination between civilian public health responses, the military and the police, and some members of the IC in the event of a bioterrorism attack (Nicoll & Murray 2002, 132). Other than the establishment of the HPA, the post-9/11 policy environment in the UK did not result in any additional significant changes to existing health security response settings within government, including in key areas such as preparedness and emergency response, which contrasts with larger politically driven and more frequent policy changes in the US, as discussed shortly.

Leaving aside the larger population and economy of the US, during the first years after 9/11 and Amerithrax, the UK government also made only modest increases in funding for countering some aspects of health security threats, risks, and hazards. For example, according to the Select Committee of Science and Development, GBP 260 million was allocated in 2003 for bio-release countermeasures in chemical, biological, radiological and nuclear (CBRN) terrorism (Jones 2005). This contrasts with an estimated US government expenditure on civilian biodefense to be around the equivalent of GBP 22 billion for the period 2001–2005, or 18 times the figure spent in 2001 (Jones 2005). Similarly, comparing the two national agencies primarily responsible for health security preparedness (the UK's HPA vs. US CDC), in 2003 the former spent GBP 160 million on bio-release countermeasures compared to the latter's total budget of USD 6.7 billion, of which 1 billion was dedicated to biodefense (Jones 2005, 346). Furthermore, it is evident that in the early post-9/11 period, political and legal concerns in the UK were rising about a lack of an overarching institutional design for addressing health security threats, risks, and hazards. This included the previously discussed 2001–02 UK House of Commons Defence Select Committee (2002) debates about how defense and civilian personnel should work together in the event of terrorist attacks that used bioweapons.

Shortly after 9/11, the policy-making focus pivoted to a wider range of health security scenarios, including the growing belief by the Blair Labour Government that terrorists would use WMDs to attack the UK, and an increasingly greater conviction that rogue states would use bioweapons. In particular, Iraq was endorsed by the UK Cabinet as an immediate threat to the UK and its allies due to its previous documented track record in the production of WMD (Chilcot 2016). Almost immediately from 2002, the principal policy focus on health security was directed at the threat of Iraq, rather than terrorists using bioweapons on UK soil, infectious diseases or biosecurity. This served to reinforce a disjuncture between international and domestic policy preparedness against a broader range of health security threats risks and hazards. It also meant that the UK lacked a comprehensive health security policy describing how all major stakeholders, including public health and national security intelligence agencies, could collaborate on a larger range of health security threats, risks, and hazards. In stock with the US Bush Administrations' policy to initially contain then enact regime change in Iraq through coalition military action, in early 2002, the Blair government in Cabinet endorsed the view that Iraq still had WMDs, including nuclear weapons, and was determined to develop them. Earlier in 2001, the UK's Joint Intelligence Committee had assessed that it was likely Iraq was producing chemical and biological agents and longer-range missiles capable of delivering them (Chilcot 2016,

43). Though as the Report of the Iraq Inquiry led by Lord Chilcott revealed, the extent of evidence and intelligence for Iraq's WMD capability was unclear and 'intelligence and assessments were used to prepare material to be used to support Government statements in a way which conveyed certainty without acknowledging the limitations of the intelligence' (Chilcot 2016, 43).

In the post-Iraq War period, UK governments did start to turn their attention to a broader (non-military) range of health security threats, risks, and hazards including infectious diseases. Sir David Omand a former Director of UK SIGINT agency GCHQ and Intelligence and Security Coordinator during the Blair Government declared in a recent article that after 9/11 in his words 'flu pandemics' 'occupied the top right-hand corner of the strategic notice risk matrix — of all the threats and risks, it posed the most lethal potential combination of impact and probability' (Omand 2020). In the few years before the COVID-19 pandemic, as McMullen notes, 'there was a greater political commitment and resourcing to UK contributions to global health security' and a 'growing centralised role of the National Security Council in health security threats, risk and hazards' targeted both domestically and internationally (McMullen 2020). This broader policy focus on health security was beyond its traditional, more narrowly focused interpretations such as WMD or bio-terrorism and can be seen in a few pre- and early COVID-19 initiatives by the UK government. A key example was the 2018 Biological Security Strategy (Bowsher et al. 2020; Cabinet Office 2018). The Strategy was a significant pre-Covid policy landmark attempting to explain the role all government agencies (public health and security) may play in managing domestic and global health security threats, risks and hazards. It adopted a relatively comprehensive four-pillar approach (understand, prevention, detection, and respond).

While it mentioned the role of intelligence agencies in the collection of information to understand risks and the role of the Ministry of Defence in understanding attribution, the document was largely vague on the general types of mandates the UK IC might play in these areas (Cabinet Office 2018). Other than briefly stating that a 'cross-departmental governance board' will oversee cross-agency activities in the strategy, the document did not explain how inevitable governance tensions will be resolved between activities deemed 'cross-departmental' vs. those which are the responsibility of existing departments and how overlaps might be managed (Cabinet Office 2018). A small qualitative study interviewing 12 senior UK leaders in global health, development, and foreign policy during 2017 reinforced this lack of clarity around the pre-COVID governance of health security in the UK. The interviewees noted the national security council in the Cabinet Office was nominally the lead on the health security agenda; however, there did not appear to be a common strategy or policy to bring cross-sector collaboration between public health, foreign policy, or national security agencies (McMullen 2020). While the rhetoric of 2018 Biological Security Strategy suggested that the UK government was finally going to address a range of health security threats/risks/hazards from a comprehensive health and security perspective, the strategy soon stalled.

A scheduled parliamentary inquiry on biological security was cancelled in 2019 as Brexit and a general election loomed, which as Bowsher et al. (2020, 3) noted 'resulted in a total arrest of central planning to build on the recommendations of the Biological Security Strategy.' Policy engagement with health security issues as a priority to be holistically operationalized across the health and security sectors stalled as the UK became mired in leaving the EU and domestic politics. Several political and bureaucratic actions in reaction to the pandemic exacerbated a lack of policy engagement by reinforcing poor historical governance challenges in managing health security and increasing a lack of preparedness. Significant bureaucratic transformation, such as the replacement of Public Health England with the National Institute for Health Protection in 2020, was implemented during a health security crisis. The Joint Biosecurity Centre, which was previously housed in the Institute, was modelled after the intelligence community's Joint Terrorism Advisory Centre (JTAC), which provides the government with threat-level warnings on terrorism. In the case of the Joint Biosecurity Centre, its function was to provide threat levels on COVID-19. These changes were on top of other stand-up policy advisory groups such as the Scientific Advisory Group for Emergencies (SAGE), which also had a role in providing senior policymakers with advice on managing the pandemic. While it is not the focus of this chapter to provide a detailed analysis of how these 'on the fly' policy reforms resulted in a suboptimal response to the pandemic (see, for example, Chapter 5 for further analysis), the renewed policy engagement and subsequent bureaucratic reforms in response to the COVID pandemic were criticized for providing the government with a very narrow 'epidemiological modelling approach' to formulate policy responses without a broader consideration (Bowsher et al. 2020). This lack of coherent governance and the government's policy response in responding to COVID-19 including how UK national security intelligence agencies may most effectively play their role reduced further the preparedness, management, and resilience against COVID-19.

At the time of writing, all 'Five Eyes' governments, including in the UK, have moved out of the acute and emergency phase of the pandemic. They are issuing a range of policy declarations, strategies, and statements to learn the lessons of COVID-19, particularly aimed at national preparedness and readiness from threat/risk/hazard detection to recovery. The former Johnson government's 2021 Integrated Review of Security, Defence, Development and Foreign Policy (herein, the Integrated Review) demonstrates the government's clear intention to better resilience post-COVID, including health security (Cabinet Office 2021). The Integrated Review says its first goal is to build national resilience, which it argues, 'is the product of effective and trusted governance, government capabilities, social cohesion and individual and business resilience' (Cabinet Office 2021, 87). However, previous policy declarations that stalled without delivering results contained similar rhetoric, such as calls to establish 'a whole of society' and 'one health' approaches to resilience' and integrate 'national security with economic health, environmental policy.' Unsurprisingly, the Integrated Review was short on detail on how effective governance will be implemented to build national resilience in health security (Cabinet Office 2021, 88).

Additionally, the lack of an integrated health security approach has also extended into the UK's forward-looking efforts evaluating national health security readiness and response. In December 2022, the UK Government appointed Baroness Heather Hallet to lead an independent inquiry into the UK's response to COVID-19, including its preparedness, interventions, and lessons that should be learnt from past policy-related investigations (Cabinet Office 2022). The Inquiry website does not specifically mention whether Britain's national security and intelligence community will be invited to testify before hearings, which commenced in June 2023 (Cabinet Office 2022). The Hallet Inquiry hearings are ongoing and not expected to be completed until around July 2025. Finally, in June 2023 the UK government launched the new Biological Security strategy which appears to be the government's latest attempt to understand emerging health security threats, risks and hazards, and fuse public health information and national security intelligence to 'enhance situational awareness and to strengthen collective decision-making and improve the effectiveness of decision-making' (Cabinet Office 2023, 23). The new biological security strategy devotes an entire section on 'leadership, governance and coordination' and includes measures such as installing a lead minister and an overall senior responsible officer (most likely the deputy national security advisor) to oversee its implementation (Cabinet Office 2023, 56). The strategy goes much further in describing how various aspects of the UK's IC might be involved in and work with public health and other important stakeholders, but time will tell if it can fully address the many historic governance and leadership challenges underscored in previous pre-COVID political and policy described above. Chapter 5 (Bowsher) will investigate whether the UK and other 'Five Eyes' governments are currently learning the lessons of COVID-19, which, as we suggest in this chapter, are lessons that have *not* been learned cumulatively since 9/11.

United States

Similar to several UK governments from 1945 to the end of the Cold War the primary policy focus of several US administrations was 'state-based biological weapons programmes' with the former Soviet Union's extensive bioweapons program being the primary concern (Walsh 2018, 25). The US had a large bioweapons program that weaponized Bacillus anthracis, Francisella tularensis, Brucella suis, and Venezuelan equine encephalitis virus (VEE), amongst others (Walsh 2018). The US Army's Directorate of Biological Operations at Pine Bluff Arsenal (Arkansas) had a capacity of 86,000 gallons though there also were other large plants at Vigo in Indiana (Regis 1999). The history of the US bioweapons program, as well as its Soviet equivalent, which lasted until the end of the Cold War, is remarkable in that it demonstrates how breakthroughs in post-war microbiology could be rapidly industrialized to develop major bioweapons programs. However, a full examination of these programs is beyond the scope of this chapter. For readers looking for in-depth coverage of these programs, Regis (1999) and Kenneth Alibek's interview with Tucker (1999) provide helpful overviews. By the late 1960s, US President Nixon announced a termination of the offensive American bioweapons program. As discussed above, in the examination of important UK health security policy milestones, policymakers in London and Washington concluded that the increasing capacity of atomic weapons provided a more reliable offensive option than a bacterial bomb (Balmer 2002).

There was a shift in policy circles in Washington based on a mixture of technical, economic, political, and legal considerations about how immediate a threat state-based biological weapons were (Balmer 2002). While US policymakers may have been scaling back the resources for offensive biological weapons, they began to express similar concerns to their UK counterparts during and up to the end of the Cold War about several rogue states (Iraq, Iran, Syria, and North Korea) that were seeking to develop biological weapons (Koblentz 2009; Spiers 2010). Out of all of these, Iraq seemed to be the one that the US intelligence community knew the most about. Iraq showed an early interest (as far back as 1974) in developing biological weapons for their strategic deterrent value (Koblentz 2009). By 1990, the Hussein regime had tested and weaponized anthrax and botulinum toxin using 400-kilogram aerial bombs and Al Hussein warheads. Though these were thankfully not very efficient at disseminating biological weapons and the regime never produced dried, powder agents, which could have covered greater differences and potentially had more lethality (UNMOVIC 2007). By the end of the first Gulf War in 1991, as UN weapon teams moved into Iraq, the Iraqi regime's offensive BW program was destroyed by inspectors including its bulk supply of biological agents and munitions (Koblentz 2009).

During the mid-1990s, policymakers started to shift their focus again from historical and traditional notions of biothreats (state-sponsored conventional biological weapons programs) to the use of biological agents by non-state actors—primarily terrorists (Koblentz 2009). Several events raised concerns in Washington about the threat from non-state actors using bioweapons. The fall of the Soviet Union and the risk of its former bio-weapons scientists becoming 'guns for hire' to terrorists, the 1995 Aum Shinrikyo subway attack in Tokyo (Leitenberg 2001; Rosenau 2001), the 1993 attack on the World Trade Center in New York and the 1996 terrorist attack in Oklahoma city all made clear to policymakers, Gronvall argues, that the United States was vulnerable to terrorism. The implication is that some groups might use biological weapons (Russell & Gronvall 2012). Further, the 9/11 attacks on the US combined with some senior officials wrongly assuming there was a link between Iraq's Hussein regime and Al Qaeda (with the former even potentially supplying the latter with bioweapons) consolidated the Bush Administrations' threat perception of health security as a narrow band of rogue state-sponsored WMD and bioterrorism from non-state actors like Al Qaeda. As previously noted, the faulty and politicized intelligence that Iraq still possessed WMD, as well as the scant evidence of US soldiers discovering technical documents and equipment in a 'biological weapons laboratory' under construction near Kandahar, underscored for the Bush Administration Iraq and Al Qaeda had both the intent and likely the increasing capability to develop biological weapons (Pita & Gunaratna 2009; Tenet 2007).

The Bush Administration also expressed concerns publicly that advances in biotechnology and life sciences would result in the creation by adversaries of new novel bioweapons that would require 'new detection methods, preventive measures and treatments' (Spiers 2010, 156). In April 2005, the Administration said:

These trends increase the risk of surprise. Anticipating such threats through intelligence efforts is made more difficult by the dual-use nature of biotechnologies and infrastructure and the likelihood that adversaries will use denial and deception to conceal their illicit activities.

(Spiers 2010, 156)

Even after faulty intelligence on Iraq's WMD possession led to the US-led invasion of Iraq in 2003, other senior US legislators maintained that the threat from biological weapons was growing and that genetic modification techniques would 'allow the creation of even worse biological weapons' (Robb et al. 2005, 34). Another important aspect of this issue is that there were differences of opinion within the US intelligence community and among biodefense experts on how significant the level of threat and capabilities Al Qaida posed in bioweapons development pre-2001 and post the invasion of Afghanistan (Leitenberg 2005; The Commission on the Intelligence Capabilities of the United States Regarding Weapons of Mass Destruction 2005). Such policy pronouncements during 1999–2009 were not consistently based on 'sophisticated threat assessments' and for many researchers in the field were 'systematically and deliberately being exaggerated' (Leitenberg 2005). In contrast to the low-grade capabilities to weaponize dangerous pathogens by terrorist groups such as Aum Shinrikyo and Al Qaeda, the September/October Anthrax letter attacks allegedly orchestrated by microbiologist Bruce Ivins in 2001 may have vindicated the rhetoric that 'bioterrorism' was a significant threat and needed to be invested in accordingly. However, that attack vector was from a domestic scientist rather than a foreign novice terrorist was likely a surprise to many in the Administration (The US Department of Justice 2010; Walsh 2018). In short, throughout at least the first term of the Bush Administration, the White House was fixing its narrow health security policy in terms of rhetoric around the prism of biodefense against rogue states like Iraq and terrorist groups (Al Qaeda) rather than an integrated one health approach that looked more comprehensively across the one health spectrum.

The policy focus and legislation enacted by the Bush Administration during this time underscore a narrower interpretation of health security threats, risks, and hazards to one marked by domestic biodefense. For example, as noted by Koblentz 'up to 40% (or 23.6 billion) was spent on biodefense (from 2001–2009) for research and development of countermeasures, diagnostics and sensors, and the construction of high containment labs (Koblentz 2012, 136–137). It's clear some US intelligence agencies, including the FBI and DHS, had a role in helping support such biodefense measures (Walsh 2018). For example, the Biowatch Program established in 2003 by the Bush Administration and managed by DHS designed to provide a nationwide aerosol detection system for biothreat agents initially for 30 of the most populous cities in the United States is one of many biodefense measures employed during the Bush years. The effectiveness of Biowatch has been limited however since its initial implementation due to a range of technical, communication, and funding reasons. For a detailed analysis see, for example, Homeland Security (2018); Currie (2016), Government Accountability Office (2014), and Willman (2017).

This domestic biodefense focus was also demonstrated in landmark legislation passed during the Bush Administration. For example, the 2002 Public Health Security and Bioterrorism Preparedness and Response Act set in motion many useful and important planks for protecting and preparing for bioterrorism acts and other health emergencies. These included increased funding for the CDC, security vetting for those with access to select agents and further research to detect biological events of concern. Nonetheless, the new legislation was largely devoid of how the intelligence community would become involved in these and other related activities described in the Act. Section 108 refers to the establishment of a working group on bioterrorism and other public emergencies to work on a series of recommendations across federal, state, and local government to prepare and respond to such threats. The Act mentions the role in such a group by the Director CIA, Secretary of Defence and Energy. All three are heads of IC agencies yet the act remains vague on the specific mandate these and other IC agencies should bring in a broad (unclassified) sense and how they might work with the US Health and Human Services and Department of Agriculture to bring about key recommendations (A to G) listed in the legislation (House of Energy and Commerce 2001).

Increasingly from 9/11, there was another cluster of health security threats risks and hazards which did not sit neatly under existing classifiers of 'biodefense' or 'bioterrorism' but also began to capture the attention of scholars and policymakers post 9/11. 'Bio-crime' was one such area, though novel infectious diseases of global significance grabbed the most focus of policymakers post-9/11 (Walsh 2018). Many of these, such as the 2003 SARS outbreak, the 2009 H1N1 influenza pandemic, the 2014 West African Ebola outbreak and the 2015 expansion of the Zika virus into South America were traditionally viewed as public health emergencies given that they were the result of natural causes and not the intentional or malevolent actions of threat actors (Walsh 2018). Nevertheless, all these cases had wider impacts beyond public health. They showed how the pathogen involved was zoonotic (i.e., could move from one species to another), and each impacted significantly on the global economy and wealth of nations. For example, SARS forced the closure of airports, reduced global travel, and resulted in increased sick days in many countries. In the broadest sense of what 'national security' means, such pandemics, particularly zoonotic ones including COVID-19, can have profound impacts on the political, social, and economic resilience of nations.

As a result of some of these natural pandemics since 9/11, successive US administrations (like other 'Five Eyes governments in Australia, Canada, New Zealand, and the UK) implemented several policy initiatives that included a broader focus and inclusion of other non-bio-terror threats and risks such as pandemics. In the case of the US, biodefense was the main focus during the first term of the Bush Administration and 'initiatives to manage global health issues were kept largely separate… Such policy separation impacted the way the intelligence community was tasked and how it worked with the public health agencies also working on bio-risks and threats' (Walsh 2018, 67).

In contrast to the Bush years, the incoming Obama Administration placed a greater emphasis on linking traditional biodefense threats with global health security risks such as pandemics and infectious diseases. Obama's National 2009 Strategy for Countering Biological Threats underscored that global health security capacity building, dual-use research, biosafety, WMD, and state-sponsored bioweapons programs should be addressed in tandem by all stakeholders. This meant that there was a role for national security agencies in assisting with global health security issues such as pandemics, as well as the traditional responses to domestic biodefense issues. The Strategy also made clear that there needed to be a significant increase and depth in partnerships including information sharing between health and security communities to achieve its objectives (The White House 2009). Health security threats and risks were already on the IC's radar in various intelligence assessments, for example, Director of National Intelligence (2008). Additionally, in 2007 the DNI established the Biological Sciences Expert Group—a standing panel of non-government biologists to assist in assessing IC research in the life sciences and to review the scientific validity of intelligence assessments (Bhattacharjee 2009). In the same year, the DNI also created a national strategy for public health security (Koblentz 2012).

As early as 2005 the FBI established a program called Science and Technology Outreach (STOP) (later renamed the Biological Sciences Outreach Program) to build trust between the scientific and law enforcement communities (Dvorkin & Lanier 2010; Hummel 2017; Walsh 2018). Over the years the FBI outreach program has sponsored do-it-yourself amateur synthetic biology groups and biohacker events in collaboration with national and local FBI WMD coordinators (Wolinsky 2016). The Obama Strategy for Countering Biological Threats provided a further catalyst for various IC agencies to engage more with public health and scientific communities. The Strategy was accompanied by Presidential Policy Directive 2, which established an inter-agency process (including the DNI) for its implementation and a framework for monitoring its progress (The White House 2009). While the DNI was included, it was less clear what section within it should the DNI take the lead for implementing the Obama Strategy for Countering Biological Threats. What remained unclear was how the agency would identify IC enterprise-wide efforts to implement the Directive, including identifying budgetary and program priorities and the mechanics of coordinating with important stakeholders outside of the IC.

The Trump Administration occupied the White House before the commencement of COVID-19 in December 2019 and was in place throughout most of the pandemic's acute phase, i.e. December 2020. In 2018, two years into the administration Trump enacted a National Biodefense Strategy. The Biodefense Strategy was expected to 'promote a more efficient, coordinated, and accountable biodefense enterprise' by bringing together Defense, Health and Human Services, Homeland Security, and Agriculture to jointly develop a national biodefense strategy and an implementation plan (Homeland Security 2018). In some respects, rhetoric contained within the National Biodefense Strategy seems to go further than the previous US administration's efforts to encourage a whole-of-government approach to biodefense that would include medical, public, animal and plant health, emergency response, scientific and technical, law enforcement, defense, and security and intelligence. The Strategy sought to address the existing 'fragmentation throughout the complex inter-agency, intergovernmental and intersectoral biodefense enterprise' (U.S. Government Accountability Office 2020, 9). It was aimed at (1) assessing enterprise-wide threats, (2) determining optimal biodetection technologies, (3) building and maintaining emerging infectious disease surveillance, (4) establishing situational awareness and data integration, and (5) enhancing lab safety and security (U.S. Government Accountability Office 2020, 9). Several goals were mentioned in the strategy, including Goal 1 Risk Awareness, which made clear that national bio-risk decision-making needed to be informed by intelligence, forecasting, and risk assessment. Goal 1 also required 'further enhancement of intelligence and analysis activities' but failed to mention which agencies within the IC should be responsible for these activities or who should take the lead (Homeland Security 2018, 6–9).

The National Biodefense Strategy was accompanied in 2018 by the Presidential Memorandum on the Support for National Biodefense/National Security Presidential Memorandum-14 (NSPM-14): This memorandum was issued to support the National Biodefense Strategy and provided the governance arrangements to implement it. Specifically, the memorandum established two governing bodies—the Biodefense Steering Committee (chaired by the Secretary of Health and Human Services) and included the Secretaries of State, Defense, Agriculture, Veteran Affairs, Homeland Security and the Administrator of the EPA. The Steering Committee's role was to provide the strategic oversight and leadership of the National Biodefense Strategy. However, it did not include senior leadership from the US IC such as the Director of National Intelligence and their participation was only on an as-required basis, which we argue was a misstep (Homeland Security 2018). The other governance instrument was the Biodefense Coordination Team, which consisted of senior officers from the above-mentioned agencies including some input from the ODNI that provided the day-to-day functions to assist the Biodefense Coordination Team in monitoring the Strategy (Homeland Security 2018).

In a 2020 testimony before the Committee on Oversight and Reform, the Directors of Homeland Security and Justice and Health Care observed that the early implementation of the strategy had three large challenges: (1) difficulties in adopting new procedures, (2) guidance on methods for data analysis, and (3) roles and responsibilities for joint decision-making (U.S. Government Accountability Office 2020). A GAO review report two years into the implementation of the Biodefense Strategy listed similar challenges and many more. Additional challenges included staffing and organizational resources limitations to identify priority strategy areas such as identifying and documenting biodefense programs across government, a lack of capabilities to bring in expertise outside of government (e.g. private sector) where most of the biodefense expertise is located and a lack of agreement on how agencies would jointly identify and support enterprise-wide biodefense priorities rather than those at the agency level (GAO 2020, 20–30). The review report completed by the GAO concluded that the 'implementation process required attention including from stakeholders outside the Biodefense Steering Committee such as the National Security Council Staff, OMB and the Congress' (U.S. Government Accountability

Office, 2020, 29). In particular, the GAO review noted how 'staff turnover within the NSC contributed to a lack of consistent leadership from the White House, which created a lapse in momentum and disrupted the implementation process' (U.S. Government Accountability Office 2020, 29).

Shortly after the February 2020 GAO report into the implementation of the national biodefense strategy was released COVID-19 reached the US and any ongoing implementation of the Biodefense Strategy was sidelined as the Trump White House confronted the COVID-19 pandemic. The many good ideas contained within the NSPM-14 and the National Biodefense Strategy for creating an enterprise-wide risk management approach to biodefense stalled as a more disorganized and politicized process defined the White House's response to the pandemic (Alexander et al. 2022; Parker & Stern 2022; Rutledge 2020).

On the point of politicization, there are a few key examples that became evident during the Trump Administration. For example, in 2016, the Obama administration developed a response plan based on lessons learnt from Ebola and Zika, a document titled 'Playbook for Early Response to High-Consequence Emerging Infectious Disease Threats and Biological Incidents.' The document included risk considerations about novel coronaviruses and offered a plan for a coordinated national response to a potential epidemic; in 2020, the Trump administration dismissed the advice of the outgoing administration, only to blame it once the pandemic swept the US (Yamey & Gonsalves 2020). We also saw how politicized during the Trump Administration the issue of tasking the IC to find the origins of COVID-19 became (Walsh et al. 2023).

In summary, several key initiatives from successive US administrations showed a narrow and somewhat fragmented approach. Biodefense political and policy responses focused almost exclusively on traditional state and non-state actor bio threats. In the Bush years in particular, zoonotic diseases were often cast as requiring public health or biosecurity responses not national security ones and were often running in parallel with policy initiatives in the biodefense domain led by the military or in some cases agencies within the intelligence community. The Obama and later Trump Administration's strategy around health security do show efforts to bring global health security, biodefense and biosecurity threats, risks, and hazards together. However, the net result of treating some health security threats and risks (e.g., pandemics) as a public health problem only and others (e.g., bioterrorism) as a national security threat reinforced a lack of governance, leadership, and mission integration within and across a range of health security threats, risks, and hazards.

The COVID-19 Health Security Choke Points: Preparedness, Governance, Threat Assessment, Ethics, and International Coordination

We now turn to the second section which assesses the key factors from 9/11 to the start of the COVID-19 pandemic that impacted both the UK and US ICs ability to play a consistent and coherent role in supporting the management of health security threats, risks, and hazards during this period. As noted earlier the analysis here relies on secondary data sources. A more comprehensive study of constraining political, policy, and institutional factors would only be possible with detailed interviews of a significant sample of IC personnel who have had responsibility in managing health security threats, risks, and hazards during this timeframe. This may be possible in the future and would be desirable to test the weighting we put on the significance of various factors discussed here. Currently, however, such a study is beyond the logistical possibilities of the authors. Nonetheless, there are sufficient, detailed, and quality secondary data sources in which to assess factors that were consistently at play from 9/11 up to COVID-19 that constrained both political decision-making and IC leadership's ability to develop capabilities to support the management of health security threats, risks, and hazards more effectively during this time frame.

Preparedness

COVID-19 was a large-scale test of decades of planning and preparation for such events. While all pandemic events are unique, the lessons to be learnt often fall into the same categories of prevention, preparedness, mitigation, and response. We argued above that COVID just amplified a range of legacy factors that had not been sufficiently dealt with historically in the policy, political, and institutional responses to a range of health security threats, risks, and hazards from 9/11 to the COVID pandemic.

The brief overview of both UK and US political and policy initiatives discussed above underscores that neither political rhetoric nor even preparedness equals action. This point is well illustrated by the paradox between global health preparedness and an actual response to the Covid-19 crisis. The 2019 Global Health Security Index published by the Nuclear Threat Initiative and Johns Hopkins Centre for Health Security evaluated the United States as the top country in its preparedness for prevention of the emergence or release of pathogens, early detection and reporting for epidemics of potential international concern and rapid response and mitigation of the spread of an epidemic, while noting that no country was fully prepared for an epidemic (GHS Index 2021). Other 'Five Eyes' countries were in the top five overall well-prepared scores in the index though interestingly New Zealand was ranked thirty-fifth (GHS Index 2021).

While the United States was rated as no. 1 on the Global Health Security Index, it performed worse than many other countries, including New Zealand, as noted which had been rated thirty-fifth in the world on the same index for preparedness. The Trump Administration dismissed previous preparedness plans, delayed national response, and engaged in blame rhetoric (Parker & Stern 2022; Schismenos et al. 2021; Yamey & Gonsalves 2020). In 2021, the Center for Disease Control and Prevention (CDC) reviewed its response to the COVID-19 pandemic and officially admitted that its response to both COVID-19 and monkeypox 'did not reliably meet expectations' despite the '75 years CDC and public health have been preparing for COVID-19,' triggering a major restructure (Sun & Diamond 2022).

The COVID-19 response miscoordination in the US resulted in 21% of the global infections and deaths attributed to COVID-19 (Muellbauer, Aron, Janine 2020). In contrast, New Zealand's government, despite being ranked lower in pandemic response preparedness, adopted a swift pandemic response initially focused on eliminating COVID-19 and later adopted graduated risk-informed suppression measures (Jefferies et al. 2020). These measures helped New Zealand achieve low levels of population illness disparities, a low relative disease burden, and the initial effectiveness of COVID-19 eradication (Jefferies et al. 2020). The unexpected variations in national responses highlight the importance not only of public health preparedness to contain disease, but also the importance of political and institutional coordination.

Governance

The history of political and institutional coordination of health security threats, risks, and hazards from 9/11 to COVID-19 demonstrates that the effectiveness of preparedness, mitigation, and response measures is dependent on a variety of elements, the most important of which is undoubtedly robust governance. Governance also influences other themes we have discovered having an impact on health security preparedness, such as resolving legal and ethical challenges, strategic vs. operational planning, risk, threat/hazard methodologies and institutional cultures. Good governance means public health, national security agencies, and other stakeholders all know what their mission, mandates, and accountability points are in large bureaucratic environments at national, regional, and local levels.

Governance in the intelligence context has an external and an internal component. External governance relates to how well governments understand health security, threat risks and hazards, and the extent to which they can fund and sustain the development of evidence-based (less politicized) policy outcomes to improve preparedness, mitigation, and response (Walsh 2011). Internal governance relates to how senior leaders of public health and national security intelligence agencies can prosecute the development of strategic and operational capabilities to identify, prevent, mitigate, and respond to health security threats, risks, and hazards (Walsh 2011). Our analysis suggests that both poor internal and external governance has contributed to the inconsistent whole-of-government approaches taken to health security issues from 9/11 to the present.

While administrations in both the UK and the US have evolved in the development of strategic health security planning that includes the right kind of rhetoric of being 'one-health' or 'multi-disciplinary,' these frameworks have often failed to develop into integrated political and institutional responses to health security over time. The net result of this has contributed to a lack of preparedness to optimally manage health security threats, risks, and hazards during the period focused on in this chapter, including COVID-19. From an external governance or political standpoint, it is clear that political interests in health security-related threats, risks, and hazards have not been consistent in both the UK and the US, especially in the earlier post-9/11 period when viewed through a narrower health security prism such as 'biodefense' or 'bioterrorism.'

There are a few other factors that are related to governance which have also impacted the extent to which policymakers and ICs have engaged effectively with health security threats, risks, and hazards in recent decades. These include political-cultural differences even between the UK and the US and other 'Five Eyes' countries. COVID-19, putting aside the influences of politicization, also underscored differences between how each 'Five Eyes' country adopted public health intervention policies within the confines of their political systems. One could argue the more fractured, 'tribal,' and innate mistrust of centralized power baked into the US federal political system would not allow the same kind of federal and state cooperation seen in Australia or New Zealand when it came to prosecuting various public health orders that restricted the liberties of citizens in the earlier stages of the pandemic. In other words, the art of what is 'politically doable' in both a legislative and political sense must also be understood in the existing nation's political culture which historically may or may not facilitate rapid emergency policy measures in some liberal democratic states as was seen during COVID-19.

Narrow and sometimes fragmented policy perspectives contributed to a less holistic understanding and warning of the range of health security issues governments ideally should know about. In turn, a narrower political focus on what might be seen as more 'traditional' biothreats (e.g., WMD/CBRN and terrorism or rogue actor's use of bio-weapons) also influences how the IC leadership views the collection, analytical, and operational priorities within their agencies of health security threats, risks, and hazards. Equally, a specific narrower focus on one threat actor group (e.g., WMD by state actors) does not necessarily equip IC agencies with the relevant threat and risk methodologies to understand let alone collect relevant intelligence on CBRN terrorism, biohackers, or pandemics. This in turn compounds the ability of ICs to effectively warn decision-makers of other potentially emerging health security, threats, and risks. Both policy and IC group think can also lead to insufficient intelligence collection and assessment, which in turn leads to intelligence and policy failure either/or at the tactical and strategic levels.

The understanding and operationalizing of what constitutes a legitimate national security threat like pandemics have of course been evolving within ICs from 9/11 to COVID-19. Comments made by former distinguished IC leaders show how national security implications of once less traditional bread and butter issues for them like pandemics have now increasingly been understood as well as the role IC agencies should play in supporting government to manage them.

For example, as noted earlier, former distinguished UK IC leader Sir David Omand in a 2021 article written during COVID-19 argues that during his time in government flu pandemics were considered high-priority risks with presumably all the resource allocation that such a designation brings (Omand 2021). In the same article Omand made some suggestions on how ICs can play a greater role in health security, including building a greater capability to do so (Omand 2021).

Yet in an earlier article he had suggested that the 'assessment of disease outbreak is not the business of the intelligence community, though he said governments need warnings on these things which need to be a robust combination of intelligence and scientific assessments' (Omand 2020). Omand's 2020 comment seems to reflect a more traditional perspective on what role ICs should play in pandemics—one that some IC leaders may still share in the current post-COVID period (Walsh et al. 2023). COVID-19 will likely continue to challenge at least to some extent the longstanding organizational cultures of ICs—a culture that for decades has been built around responding to threat actors, not more amorphous risks and hazards like pandemics or climate change (Walsh et al. 2023). It is clear, however, that Omand's 2020 perspective has evolved like many IC leaders after COVID-19. Omand's earlier 2020 statement about the 'assessment of disease outbreaks' somehow not being in the lane also of national security intelligence agencies we argue is somewhat contradictory because to provide robust intelligence warning one needs IC staff who understand well both the scientific, health, and intelligence on health security and how it relates to the national security intelligence information, particularly if you are trying to build better warning systems post-COVID.

Just how many people in the IC need to have this knowledge and where located will require careful consideration post-COVID-19 by all governments and particularly the IC leadership. These issues are taken up in Chapter 8 by Vogel. It will be in part determined by budgets, IC leadership and governance, and whether political leadership expects to see more IC health security products that are multidisciplinary in nature.

Ethics

In addition to any political legal and constitutional challenges faced by political leaders in the management of health security crises like COVID-19, the history of political and policy responses to these issues also shows a series of ethical dilemmas for policymakers and ICs in what is the appropriate level of intrusion into citizen's privacy (medical history and identity-related data) and their liberty in implementing various public health orders and other non-pharmaceutical interventions.

What is clear from our survey of policy action from 9/11 to COVID-19 is that greater integration and collaboration needs to occur between public health and national security agencies particularly ways to share more rapidly data sources of relevance to the mission of both sectors. However, also as seen during the period examined in this chapter, institutionalizing cooperation between health and security agencies implies potentially a securitization of the public health area. The intended goal of linking health with security data sources is to rapidly identify and disrupt the spread of infectious diseases with the least loss of life and negative impacts on social and economic life. However, overt securitization might have unintended consequences, such as restricting the work of public health scientists (Vines 2018). Political pushes towards more securitization without clear accountability mechanisms in place might lead to populist purposes of 'political policy', where more securitization might not be required. It is therefore key that decision-makers deploy ethical considerations before melting barriers to information sharing across government jurisdictions.

Ethical practices in the expansion of increased integration continue to be a contested area. Walsh and Miller (2015), Miller et al. 2022 amongst others, for example Henschke et al. 2024, contend that intelligence studies literature has been slow in identifying ethical aspects of intelligence practice, but also critiques anti-intelligence activism that does not offer pathways to ensure national security. They argue that policy guidelines should not necessarily provide "specific 'one size fits all' policy prescriptions, but rather develop generic standards, purposes and parameters that could apply to different contexts" and propose that they should con-sider (1) methods, (2) context, and (3) targets of intelligence gathering (Walsh & Miller 2015, 348–349). Miller and Blackler (2005) expand those ideas by detailing six ethical principles that should follow:

1 Surveillance and interception are in themselves an infringement of the individual's right to privacy and should therefore be only overridden by other moral considerations, such as preserving the right to life during wartime.
2 Benefits of surveillance must intercept the costs.
3 Surveillance must be deployed only for serious crimes.
4 Reasonable suspicion/belief that a crime and/or probable cause that the indi-vidual under surveillance is intending to commit a crime.
5 No alternative feasible method should be available to obtain the information required.
6 Law enforcement must be subject to strict accountability requirements.
7 Individuals under surveillance must be informed about surveillance at the earliest time following the completion of the investigation.

Despite the complex issues surrounding the ethical expansion of public health intelligence, scholarly literature has identified some best practices in evaluating the need for intelligence and surveillance as well as their evaluation. Additionally, proactive measures of public consultation have also been engaged by some governments: in 2019, New Zealand announced an overhaul of the country's Biosecurity Act and included a formalized consultation process with Māori, industry partners, environmental groups, among other groups, as well as a plan for a period for formal public consultation (MPI 2019). Although scholars have called for increasing accountability requirements (Walsh & Miller 2015), signifi-cant concerns (e.g., the effectiveness of expanded security rights) remain unad-dressed. Seumas Miller's contribution (Chapter 7) explores these issues in detail particularly how post COVID-19 the many ethical risks emerging from the use of public health data during the pandemic and the conditions under which national security agencies may have access to it in any future health security emergencies is unresolved.

International Health Security Coordination

A final dimension to how policymakers and ICs engaged with health security threats, risks and hazards relates to the extent 'Five Eyes' states have participated in various international and multilateral health initiatives during the period studied in this chapter. While the chapter focus has been on how domestic policy initiatives in the UK and the US have impacted IC's ability to support health security, the role of international health institutions and initiatives no doubt has also impacted 'Five Eyes' countries' ability to receive, timely and accurate global health data useful to providing early warning and decision maker support. Historically, international utilization of health security intelligence faces an even larger number of challenges in working together to counter health security threats. Even when health intelligence is collected, numerous barriers exist to effectively communicating that information. For instance, during the early months of the 2014–2016 Western Africa Ebola outbreak, several factors contributed to health intelligence failure, including the Guinean government's inadequate capacity to handle the crisis, the government's inaccurate assessments of the crisis, the US embassy's failure to contextualize the risk information appropriately, and the US embassy's readiness to accept the Guinean government's assessment without question (Ostergard 2021).

At the international level, rapidly spreading infectious diseases are monitored by the Global Outbreak Alert and Response Network (GOARN), which was formed in 2000 and places the World Health Organization (WHO) at the center of network coordination. GOARN is a network of more than 250 global institutions and networks that can help respond to and deploy staff and resources (Global Outbreak Alert and Response Network, n.d.). After the 2002–2003 SARS outbreak, GOARN was linked at the international and national level: national systems were to monitor disease outbreaks national and report their data to the WHO, which could then monitor and report outbreaks as well as liaise with countries affected (Wark 2021). Equipped with the International Health Regulations that mandated outbreak reporting, GOARN was to rely on transparent national reporting and the WHO's capabilities to aggregate information internationally. To add to the information in case some countries were unable or unwilling to report outbreak data, the WHO included additional reporting from non-state sources. One of those sources was the Canadian Global Public Health Intelligence Network (GPHIN) (Government of Canada n.d.). In 2019 and 2020, however, the GPHIN failed to report on COVID-19, for reasons that were later uncovered via investigative journalism including: Canadian officials' focus redirection away from global to North American health monitoring, technological issues, budget shortfalls, restraints on internal scientific reporting, mismanagement, cessation of reporting to global instruments (Wark 2021; Government of Canada 2023). The review of GOARN is still underway (Global Outbreak Alert and Response Network, n.d.), which will determine how international health intelligence will be coordinated across the interconnected national and international levels. A broader review of the WHO's early warning capabilities has also taken place along with a range of other multi-lateral measures including potentially an international health treaty aimed at mandating greater transparency on disease outbreaks of concern by member states. These post-COVID international measures are discussed by Lentzos in Chapter 9.

Conclusion

Barriers to effective political engagement at both the domestic policy and IC institutional levels as noted above have been many and accumulated over several decades from 9/11 up to including the COVID-19 pandemic. The solutions to addressing such constraints are not straightforward both at the political, policy and IC institutional levels. The remaining chapters will pick up many of the themes identified here and examine how they might begin to be addressed. There is again, as in the past, a small window to keep policy maker's attention on health security threats, risks, and hazards in the wake of COVID-19 before it seems the inevitable disengagement on these issues begins again.

References

Alexander, M., Unruh, L., Koval, A., & Belanger, W. (2022). United States Response to the COVID-19 Pandemic, January–November 2020. *Health Economics, Policy and Law*, *17*(1), 62–75. https://doi.org/10.1017/S1744133121000116

Balmer, B. (2002). Biological Warfare: The Threat in Historical Perspective. *Medicine, Conflict and Survival*, *18*(2), 120–137. https://doi.org/10.1080/13623690208409619

Bhattacharjee, Y. (2009). Paul Keim on His Life with the FBI During the Anthrax Investigation. *Science*, *323*(5920), 1416–1416. https://doi.org/10.1126/science.323.5920.1416

Bowsher, G., Bernard, R., & Sullivan, R. (2020). A Health Intelligence Framework for Pandemic Response: Lessons from the UK Experience of COVID-19. *Health Security*, *18*(6), 435–443. https://doi.org/10.1089/hs.2020.0108

Cabinet Office (2018). *Biological Security Strategy*. www.gov.uk/government/publications/biological-security-strategy

Cabinet Office (2021). *Global Britain in a Competitive Age: The Integrated Review of Security, Defence, Development and Foreign Policy*. www.gov.uk/government/publications/global-britain-in-a-competitive-age-the-integrated-review-of-security-defence-development-and-foreign-policy

Cabinet Office (2022). *UK COVID-19 Inquiry: Terms of Reference*. www.gov.uk/government/publications/uk-covid-19-inquiry-terms-of-reference

Cabinet Office (2023). *UK Biological Security Strategy*. www.gov.uk/government/publications/uk-biological-security-strategy/uk-biological-security-strategy-html

Carus, W. S. (2017). *A Short History of Biological Warfare: From Pre-History to the 21st Century*. National Defense University Press.

Chilcot, J. (2016). *The Report of the Iraq Inquiry: Executive Summary*. https://policycommons.net/artifacts/2481047/the_report_of_the_iraq_inquiry_-_executive_summary/3503232/

Currie, C. (2016). *Biosurveillance. Ongoing Challenges and Future Consideration for DHS Biosurveillance Efforts*. www.gao.gov/products/gao-16-413t

Director of National Intelligence (2008). *Strategic Implications of Global Health*. www.dni.gov/files/documents/Special%20Report_ICA%20Global%20Health%202008.pdf

Dvorkin, D., & Lanier, W. (2010). Synthetic Bio, Meet FBIo. *The Scientist, 24*(7).

GHS Index. (2021). *2021 Global Health Security Index.* www.ghsindex.org/

Global Outbreak Alert and Response Network (n.d.). https://goarn.who.int/#topstories

Government Accountability Office (2014). Biosurveillance, Observations on the Cancellation of BioWatch Gen-3 and Future Considerations for the Program: Testimony Before the Subcommittee on Emergency Preparedness, Response, and Communications, Committee on Homeland Security, House of Representatives. www.gao.gov/assets/gao-14-267t.pdf

Government of Canada (2023). Independent Review of the Global Public Health Intelligence Network (GPHIN). www.canada.ca/en/public-health/corporate/mandate/about-agency/external-advisory-bodies/list/independent-review-global-public-health-intelligence-network.html

Government of Canada (n.d.). Global Public Health Intelligence Network. https://gphin.canada.ca/cepr/aboutgphin-rmispenbref.jsp?language=en_CA

Henschke, A., Miller, S., Alexandra, A., Walsh, P. F., & Bradbury, R. (2024). *The Ethics of National Security Intelligence Institutions: Theory and Applications* (p. 249). Taylor & Francis.

Homeland Security (2018). *The President's Biodefense Strategy.* www.dhs.gov/archive/coronavirus/presidents-biodefense-strategy

Human Security Centre (2006). *Human Security Report 2005: War and Peace in the 21st Century.* https://global.oup.com/academic/product/human-security-report-2005-9780195307399?cc=au&lang=en&

Hummel, K. (2017). A View from the CT Foxhole: Edward You, FBI Weapons of Mass Destruction Directorate, Biological Countermeasures Unit. *CTC Sentinel, 10*, 9–12.

Jefferies, S., French, N., Gilkison, C., Graham, G., Hope, V., Marshall, J., McElnay, C., McNeill, A., Muellner, P., Paine, S., Prasad, N., Scott, J., Sherwood, J., Yang, L., & Priest, P. (2020). COVID-19 in New Zealand and the Impact of the National Response: A Descriptive Epidemiological Study. *The Lancet Public Health, 5*(11), e612–e623. https://doi.org/10.1016/S2468-2667(20)30225-5

Jones, D. (2005). Structures of Bio-Terrorism Preparedness in the UK and the US: Responses to 9/11 and the Anthrax Attacks. *The British Journal of Politics and International Relations, 7*(3), 340–352. https://doi.org/10.1111/j.1467-856X.2005.00189.x

Koblentz, G. D. (2009). *Living Weapons: Biological Warfare and International Security.* Cornell University Press.

Koblentz, G. D. (2012). From Biodefence to Biosecurity: The Obama Administration's Strategy for Countering Biological Threats. *International Affairs, 88*(1), 131–148. https://doi.org/10.1111/j.1468-2346.2012.01061.x

Leitenberg, M. (2001). Who Could Use Biological Weapons?: State Proliferators and the Threat Posed by Non-State Actors. *Track Two: Constructive Approaches to Community and Political Conflict, 10*(3). https://hdl.handle.net/10520/EJC111524

Leitenberg, M. (2005). *Assessing the Biological Weapons and Bioterrorism Threat.* https://press.armywarcollege.edu/monographs/30/

McMullen, E. (2020). Governing the UK Contribution to Health Security: In Our National Interest? *Research Square.* https://doi.org/10.21203/rs.3.rs-83030/v1

Miller, S., & Blackler, J. (2005). *Ethical Issues in Policing* (1st ed.). Routledge. https://doi.org/10.4324/9781315256108.

Miller, S., Regan, M., & Walsh, P. F. (2022). *National Security Intelligence and Ethics.* Taylor & Francis.

MPI (2019). *Biosecurity Act Overhaul – Frequently Asked Questions*. Ministry of Primary Industries.www.mpi.govt.nz/dmsdocument/36174-Biosecurity-Act-Review-FAQs-18-July-2019

Muellbauer, J., & Aron, J. (2020). *Vox EU*. https://cepr.org/voxeu/columns/us-excess-mortal ity-rate-covid-19-substantially-worse-europes

Nicoll, A., & Murray, V. (2002). Health Protection – A Strategy and a National Agency. *Public Health, 116*(3), 129–137. https://doi.org/https://doi.org/10.1038/sj.ph.1900847

Omand, D. (2020). Will the Intelligence Agencies Spot the Next Outbreak? *The Article*. www.thearticle.com/will-the-intelligence-agencies-spot-the-next-outbreak

Omand, D. (2021). Natural Hazards and National Security: The COVID-19 Lessons. *PRISM, 9*(2), 2–19. www.jstor.org/stable/27008972

Ostergard, R. L. (2021). The West Africa Ebola Outbreak (2014–2016): A Health Intelligence Failure? In M. S. Goodman, J. M. Wilson, & F. Lentzos (Eds.), *Health Security Intelligence* (pp. 13–28). Routledge. https://doi.org/10.4324/9781003245483

Parker, C. F., & Stern, E. K. (2022). The Trump Administration and the COVID-19 Crisis: Exploring the Warning-Response Problems and Missed Opportunities of a Public Health Emergency. *Public Administration, 100*(3), 616–632. https://doi.org/10.1111/padm.12843

Pita, R., & Gunaratna, R. (2009). Revisiting Al-Qaida's Anthrax Program. *CTC Sentinel, 2*(5), 10–13.

Public Health Security and Bioterrorism Preparedness and Response Act of 2002, (2001).

Regis, E. (1999). *The Biology of Doom: The History of America's Secret Germ Warfare Project*. Henry Holt and Company.

Robb, C. S., Silberman, L. H., Levin, R. C., McCain, J., Rowen, H. S., Slocombe, W. B., Studeman, W. O., Vest, C. M., Wald, P., & Cutler, L. (2005). The Commission on the Intelligence Capabilities of the United States Regarding Weapons of Mass Destruction: Report to the President of the United States. Commission on Intelligence Capabilities Regarding WMD.

Rosenau, W. (2001). Aum Shinrikyo's Biological Weapons Program: Why Did It Fail? *Studies in Conflict & Terrorism, 24*(4), 289–301. https://doi.org/10.1080/1057610 0120887

Russell, P. K., & Gronvall, G. K. (2012). U.S. Medical Countermeasure Development Since 2001: A Long Way Yet to Go. *Biosecurity and Bioterrorism: Biodefense Strategy, Practice, and Science, 10*(1), 66–76. https://doi.org/10.1089/bsp.2012.0305

Rutledge, P. E. (2020). Trump, COVID-19, and the War on Expertise. *The American Review of Public Administration, 50*(6–7), 505–511. https://doi.org/10.1177/027507402 0941683

Schismenos, S., Smith, A. A., Stevens, G. J., & Emmanouloudis, D. (2021). Failure to Lead on COVID-19: What Went Wrong with the United States? *International Journal of Public Leadership, 17*(1), 39–53. https://doi.org/10.1108/IJPL-08-2020-0079

Spiers, E. (2010). *A History of Chemical and Biological Weapons*. Reaktion Books.

Sun, L. H., & Diamond, D. (2022). CDC, Under Fire, Lays Out Plan to Become More Nimble and Accountable. *The Washington Post*. www.washingtonpost.com/health/2022/08/17/walensky-revamp-cdc-culture-covid/

Tenet, G. (2007). *At the Center of the Storm*. Harper Collins.

The Commission on the Intelligence Capabilities of the United States Regarding Weapons of Mass Destruction (2005). *The Commission on the Intelligence Capabilities of the United States Regarding Weapons of Mass Destruction*. https://govinfo.library.unt.edu/wmd/about.html

The US Department of Justice (2010). *Amerithrax Investigative Summary.* www.justice.gov/archive/amerithrax/docs/amx-investigative-summary.pdf

The White House (2009). Presidential Policy Directive 2: Implementation of the National Strategy for Countering Biological Threats. https://irp.fas.org/offdocs/ppd/ppd-2.pdf

Tucker, J. B. (1999). Biological Weapons in the Former Soviet Union: An Interview with Dr. Kenneth Alibek. *The Nonproliferation Review, 6*(3), 1–10. https://doi.org/10.1080/10736709908436760

UK House of Commons Defence Select Committee (2002). *Select Committee on Defence: Sixth Report.* https://publications.parliament.uk/pa/cm200203/cmselect/cmdfence/93/9308.htm

UNMOVIC (2007). *Compendium of Iraq's Prescribed Weapons Programmes in the Chemical, Biological and Missile Areas.*

U.S. Government Accountability Office (2020). *National Biodefense Strategy: Additional Efforts Would Enhance Likelihood of Effective Implementation.* www.gao.gov/products/gao-20-273

Vines, T. (2018). Beakers and Borders: Export Controls and the Life-sciences under the Defence Trade Controls Act 2012. *Journal of law and medicine, 25*(3), 655–677. http://europepmc.org/abstract/MED/29978660

Walsh, P. (2011). *Intelligence and Intelligence Analysis.* Routledge.

Walsh, P. F. (2018). *Intelligence, Biosecurity and Bioterrorism.* Springer.

Walsh, P. F. (2020). Improving 'Five Eyes' Health Security Intelligence capabilities: leadership and governance challenges. *Intelligence and National Security, 35*(4), 586–602. https://doi.org/10.1080/02684527.2020.1750156

Walsh, P. F., & Miller, S. (2015). Rethinking 'Five Eyes' Security Intelligence Collection Policies and Practice Post Snowden. *Intelligence and National Security, 31*(3), 345–368. https://doi.org/10.1080/02684527.2014.998436

Walsh, P. F., Ramsay, J., & Bernot, A. (2023). Health Security Intelligence Capabilities Post COVID-19: Resisting the Passive "New Normal" Within the Five Eyes. *Intelligence and National Security,* 1–17. https://doi.org/10.1080/02684527.2023.2231196

Wark, W. (2021). Building a Better Global Health Security Early-Warning System Post-COVID: The View from Canada. *International Journal, 76*(1), 55–67. https://doi.org/10.1177/0020702020985227

Willman, D. (2017). Judge Bars Public from Trial Over Homeland Security Contract for Device to Detect Bioterrorism. *The Los Angeles Times.* www.latimes.com/nation/la-na-dhs-gag-order-20170911-story.html

Wolinsky, H. (2016). The FBI and Biohackers: An Unusual Relationship. *EMBO Reports, 17*(6), 793–796. https://doi.org/https://doi.org/10.15252/embr.201642483

Yamey, G., & Gonsalves, G. (2020). Donald Trump: A Political Determinant of Covid-19. *BMJ, 369,* m1643. https://doi.org/10.1136/bmj.m1643

4 Disinformation

The COVID-19 Pandemic and Beyond

Jennifer Hunt

Introduction

Disinformation has emerged as a crucial national and international security concern, topping the list of risks in the World Economic Forum's 2024 Global Risks Report (World Economic Forum 2024). From pandemics to climate change, efforts to confront global challenges are impeded by the erosion of trust in science, experts and public institutions. Instead, misinformation, disinformation and conspiracy theories – some employed as part of information warfare – pollute the information global commons, poisoning understanding and action. The COVID-19 pandemic provided a vivid demonstration of the weaponization of false information. Unscientific assertions downplayed the severity of the virus, the need for mitigation efforts, and the motive of state and public health communities. These narratives compromised mitigation efforts such as masks, lockdowns and vaccination, formed the basis of radicalization and recruitment efforts for extremist groups, boosted the political currency of malicious actors, and even promoted violence. The global reach of these narratives was accelerated by technological connectivity and their influence boosted by algorithms primed for engagement rather than accuracy. This chapter examines the role of disinformation, including cyber-enabled disinformation, during the COVID-19 pandemic and its long-term implications. While the US forms the primary case study of this analysis, both as an early hotspot of the virus, and the home of the technology platforms through which disinformation spread, the effects were felt around the world and the ramifications are global in reach.

Disinformation

A plethora of terminology abounds to describe the phenomenon of confusion over facts associated with the post-truth age, including disinformation, misinformation, fake news, alternative facts, and conspiracy theories. While each term has a particular history and connotation, all share a commonality as "problematically inaccurate language that disrupts politics, business and culture" (Jack 2017, 1). Distinguishing between the main foci of this chapter, misinformation, disinformation and conspiracy theories, is intention. In much the same way that manslaughter

DOI: 10.4324/9781003335511-6

and homicide are differentiated by intent, but not outcome (in both instances there is a dead body), misinformation and disinformation are both false information, but the former is unintentionally so. Conspiracy theories occupy a fertile middle ground – being fervently believed (and thus not intentionally false), but not rising to the level of credible evidence either. The difference is potentially important for corrective strategies. If disinformation is deliberately and knowingly false, while misinformation and conspiracy theories are still inaccurate but not intentionally so, only one is amenable to correction. Conspiracy theories act as "shortcuts to understanding" particularly in a time of rapid change. For some, the moon landing, the death of JFK, a pandemic, all being overwhelming developments that only secret cabals and government orchestration could sufficiently explain them. According to social psychologist Sander van der Linden, providing its adherents a way to satisfy their skepticism of authorities, to claim insider knowledge that makes them feel valuable, and often position themselves as part of a larger mission of good against evil (NPR 2022). In this way, conspiracy theories offer clarity and community in a time of great anxiety and turmoil, and allow the individual a way to assert control over their lives during seemingly overwhelming and random global events.

Cyber-Enabled Disinformation as Information Warfare

In security studies, disinformation and conspiracy theories have been analyzed as a tactic of hostile foreign state actors. For instance, the Soviet government promulgated conspiracy theories that the CIA was responsible for the creation of AIDS, that JFK was murdered by his own government, and called into question the integrity of elections (Rid 2020; Hunt 2021). UK intelligence regularly produced assessments of Soviet disinformation operations and evolving tactics from forgeries (deep fakes) (Evans and Novak 1979) and conspiracy theories (UK Foreign Office and Foreign and Commonwealth Office 1966).[1] More recently, China and Iran have been accused of sowing confusion about COVID-19 as a means of great power competition.

In particular, security scholars and public health researchers have documented ongoing cyber-enabled disinformation campaigns around public health issues. A 2018 study examined the role of hostile foreign actors on social media platforms in undermining trust in vaccines, with Russian bots and trolls promoting confusion and discord. Broniatowski et al. (2018, 1370) concluded that Russian "accounts masquerading as legitimate users create false equivalency, eroding public consensus on vaccination." In 2020, reports by the European Commission and the US State department found that foreign actors, led by Beijing, Moscow and Tehran had carried out campaigns through social media aimed at stoking confusion about the COVID-19 pandemic and undermining state responses. Kremlin-linked sites boosted conspiracy theories that allege COVID-19 was a bioweapon, that billionaire Bill Gates is plotting to use the pandemic as an excuse to microchip people, and that plans for the vaccine are a well-orchestrated money grab by pharmaceutical companies (US State Department 2020). As some of these efforts predate COVID-19, they are likely to continue beyond it. But why?

Scholars argue that disinformation is best understood as a campaign, a suite of information actions, deployed to mislead for a strategic, political purpose (Starbird, Arif and Wilson 2019, 127). A former Soviet disinformation officer defines disinformation as "a carefully constructed false message leaked to an opponent's communication system in order to deceive the decision-making elite or the public" (Bittman 1985, 49). One of those tactics is to erode trust and credibility. The purpose is to create doubt, about facts and their sources, thus the threshold of success is not necessarily to convince but to confuse. Together these activities are known in security circles as Russian Active Measures (Watts 2017).

Active Measures

- Create general distrust or confusion over information sources by blurring the lines between fact and fiction
- Foment and exacerbate divisive political fissures
- Undermine citizen confidence in democratic governance
- Erode trust between citizens and elected officials and their institutions

The most comprehensive report on the tactics, methods and goals of disinformation campaigns were released by the US Senate Intelligence Committee. Over four volumes of their investigation of Russian Interference in the US 2016 election, these reports confirmed the cyber tools used by Russia including algorithmically targeted propaganda and disinformation campaigns launched over social media designed to rupture civil society (US SSCI 2019). The documents detail the Kremlin's strategic disinformation narratives around voter fraud in order to erode trust in electoral infrastructure and democratic processes, a narrative boosted starting in 2012, when Kremlin-aligned *Russia Today* (*RT)* ran regular segments alleging US election fraud, contending US election results cannot be trusted and do not reflect the popular will (US Director of National Intelligence 2017). This narrative, combined with a Supreme Court decision dismantling anti-discrimination provisions of the Voting Rights Act (1965) in 2013 (Condon 2013), later formed the foundation for "stolen election" narratives which emboldened thousands of people to convene at the US Capitol building threatening to kill lawmakers who certified the election (Hunt 2021). In a demonstration of the overlap of these two disinformation narratives, a speaker at the DC rally the night before the January 6 attack on the Capitol told attendees during one of the largest death tolls of the pandemic that COVID-19 was a hoax, encouraging the gathered crowd to, "Go hug somebody. Go ahead and spread it out, mass spreader. It's a mass spreader event!" (Moye 2021). An examination of specific COVID-19 disinformation narratives that would incite such behaviour is useful to identify patterns and impacts for the rest of the chapter.

COVID-19 False Narratives

As Jonathan Swift wrote, "Falsehood flies, and the Truth comes limping after it, so that when men come to be undeceived, it is too late" (Swift 1710). While scientists and researchers methodically gathered and analyzed data, disinformation was already on the march, spreading and mutating rapidly both online and off. False information coalesced around several categories including: origin of the virus, its severity, the role of institutions, mitigation efforts (lockdowns, masks), and vaccines. A brief sample is below, though specific narratives were adapted to local audiences.

Categories:

- Origin: Chinese-engineered bioweapon
- Severity: Hoax, "Just the flu" Mortality exaggerated or lethally designed population cull
- Institutions: Unprepared to active part of Deep State or globalist WHO/UN/WEF plot

Mitigation strategies:

- Lockdowns: Form of tyranny, orchestrated attack on economy to undermine Trump's re-election chances
- Masks: Ineffective to actively harmful to "God's breathing system"
- Vaccine: Unnecessary, extortion, or control and tracking mechanism using 5G

Using this list, it is easy to see how these narratives fit within a broader pattern of disinformation to "foment distrust, destabilize institutions, defame opponents and delegitimize sources of knowledge such as science and journalism" (Sinclair 2023). Ilya Yablokov (2015, 302) argues that narratives such as disinformation and conspiracy theories function to "unite audiences as 'the people' against 'the other' represented by a secretive power bloc." In this narrative, vaccines, masks and social distancing requirements are subjugation of "the people" rather than reasonable measures to limit the spread of a contagious virus. Thus, the people may rationally resist these attacks on their liberty with force, if necessary. Where these measures are the advice of the scientific elite "The Other," those prestigious institutions such as the Centers for Disease Control and Prevention (CDC), World Health Organization (WHO), or United Nations (UN), now themselves constitute a potential threat.

These narratives had several immediate impacts on the COVID-19 response, and potentially more longer-term ramifications.

1 Undermining of mitigation efforts such as masks and lockdowns, as well as vaccines
2 Politicization of scientific institutions, practitioners and researchers
3 Directing extremist-fueled violence towards above targets
4 Boosting political campaigns of conspiratorial actors

Undermining Pandemic Response

By 2021, the US had lost 1% of its total population, surpassing World War II and the 1918 Influenza Pandemic death tolls. Despite a relatively small portion of global population (5%), the US at one point represented more than 25% of global cases and by 2024 exceeded a COVID-19 death toll of more than 1 million. The *Lancet* article identified the US as having the fourth highest global number of COVID-19 orphans (Hillis et al. 2021). These numbers demonstrate in part the toll of disinformation in politicizing the pandemic response and undermining public trust in scientific institutions and practitioners.

During the pandemic and its aftermath, conspiracy theories regarding the viruses' origin and severity, the need and efficacy of public health responses and mitigation efforts, and the role of officials and global institutions was spread through social media to traditional outlets and even political actors. Repeatedly, the US administration under President Trump was accused of spreading misinformation (Saletan 2020). Surveys, protests and uptake rates of mitigation efforts provide potentially useful indicators of the success of these narratives. For instance, a July 2020 PEW Report found that those who rely most on Trump for COVID-19 news and information were more likely to believe the conspiracy theory that the outbreak was planned by powerful people (Mitchell et al. 2020). Studies also attempted to measure in real time the impact of certain news sources such as television and radio programs on their audiences' willingness to take action to protect themselves and others against Covid-19.

In one study, Jamieson and Albarracin found that people who received their information from mainstream print such as the *New York Times*, and broadcast outlets such as *NBC* tended to have an accurate assessment of the severity of the pandemic and their risks of infection. However, consumers of conservative sources such as Fox News and Rush Limbaugh were more likely to believe conspiracy theories, including that the Chinese government had created the virus, and that the US Centers for Disease Control and Prevention had exaggerated the pandemic threat to "damage the Trump Presidency". Across radio and television, conservative media undermined health communication on the lethality of the virus and the efficacy of mitigation efforts. As detailed in Ricardson (2020), Rush Limbaugh described mask wearers as "freaks" and encouraging young adults to disregard lockdowns and rely on herd immunity. Consequently, a Pew research study found the partisan divide over COVID-19 widened as the pandemic progressed. Between April and June 2020, the percentage of Republicans who said that the coronavirus was "overblown" actually increased (Mitchell et al. 2020).

These messages encouraged audience non-participation in mitigation efforts to disastrous impact. Studies estimate that in the US, 318,000 COVID-19 deaths could have been prevented if those individuals had been vaccinated (Brown University 2022). Misinformation and disinformation about COVID-19 vaccines has been estimated to have cost the US at least 50 million per day in 2021 in direct costs from hospitalization, long-term illness, lives lost and missed workdays (Bruns et al. 2021).

Disinformation was most effective when spread by groups with a high degree of social trust. In the US, this includes the military, law enforcement and officers of the court. Research demonstrates that cyber-enabled disinformation has been microtargeted to these groups, some successfully. Even after COVID-19 rocketed to become the main cause of death for law enforcement in the United States in 2020, police unions in New York, Chicago and Seattle fiercely opposed vaccine mandates (NBC News 2021). In other cases, impersonation of high-value messengers was used. Sock puppet accounts impersonating well-respected social actors such as veterans' groups, were created on social media sites to sow disinformation and other narratives, tactics which were previously demonstrated in foreign interference in the 2016 US Presidential election (Shane 2019).

The most vivid demonstration of the reach and impact of disinformation campaigns was armed demonstrators invading legislative buildings to stop elected officials from passing pandemic response measures. When armed demonstrators defied state issued stay-at-home orders by gathering illegally in front of courthouses and state legislatures, then-President Trump encouraged their actions. In April 2020, Trump tweeted to his 80 million followers, "Liberate Michigan! Liberate Virginia! Liberate Minnesota! They are trying to take your Second Amendment!" (Trump 2020). Shortly thereafter in Michigan, the governor was targeted for kidnapping, trial and potential execution by a militia group. A total of 14 participants were eventually charged with federal- and state-level domestic terrorism offenses (Clifford 2021). Across the US, demonstrators carrying tactical weapons and wearing military style gear convened at the personal residences of policymakers, health officials and judges. At the Kentucky governor's mansion, one such group gathered for the "Patriot 2nd Amendment rally" strung up an effigy of the governor with sign "Sic semper tyrannis" [Thus Always to Tyrants] around his neck. In Illinois, anti-lockdown demonstrators used Nazi slogans such as "Work Makes You Free" to intimidate the Jewish governor, a tactic which drew the rebuke of the Auschwitz Museum itself, whose verified account posted on May 2, ""Arbeit macht frei" [Work makes you free] was a false, cynical illusion the SS gave to prisoners of #Auschwitz. Those words became one of the icons of human hatred. It's painful to see this symbol instrumentalized & used again to spread hate. It's a symptom of moral & intellectual degeneration" (Auschwitz Museum 2020).

Well before a vaccine became available, disinformation was rampant regarding its necessity and its side effects. Prevalent were myths that the vaccine negatively affecting fertility in women and vaccines altering the genetic makeup of recipients or even offering futuristic side effects such as wireless 5G. Messaging was multimodal, with memes used to attract younger audiences using humor and sarcasm. A study found that anti-vaccination memes employed active measures tactics by regularly vilifying government and social institutions as politically compromised or corrupt, and merely using vaccines as a form of state surveillance, control or profit (Baker and Walsh 2024). According to an August 2020 Gallup poll, more than one-third of Americans said they wouldn't get vaccinated when it becomes available (O'Kefee 2020). Meanwhile, successful mitigation efforts in countries like Australia were portrayed as "tyranny," with one US Republican governor calling on the US review diplomatic ties (Wilson 2021). In their stead, dangerous "remedies" were peddling as cures. As Ferreira Caceres et al. (2022, 263) note, "misleading information also target[ed] beliefs for management and treatment — the consumption of alcohol, cow excrements, cow urine, colloidal silver, teas, and essential oils have all been associated with curing COVID-19 infection." Disinformation then, sought to influence people to disregard the public health emergency, and avoid taking action to protect themselves and others. In future, anti-vaccination messaging could degrade support for other types of immunizations including childhood vaccinations, on which herd immunity depends.

Politicization of Scientific Institutions, Researchers and Practitioners

Disinformation narratives around the pandemic called into question the integrity and independence of key public health institutions such as the World Health Organisation as well as health practitioners, scientists and researchers. Then-President Trump ordered a halt to the WHO funding claiming a virus "cover up" and formally withdrew the United States from the organization (reinstated by Biden the following year). These narratives drove harassment campaigns and protests against healthcare institutions and personnel. The most significant and frequently reported attacks on healthcare related to COVID-19 included threats, physical assaults and heavy weapon attacks at hospitals and health centers (WHO 2020). During the first wave of COVID-19 more than 30 senior health officials across 13 US States resigned, retired or were dismissed from their post, due to violent harassment, strain or political clashes (Mossburg 2020). Though applauded as heroes at the start of the pandemic, frontline nurses have been the target of abuse and intimidation leading to retention problems in the profession. Nurses have noted that "people accuse us of giving their loved one something else so that they would die and we could report it as Covid. We heard it more than once that we were fudging the numbers, or we were killing people on purpose to make Covid look like it was worse than it was, or to make it look real when it wasn't" (Reeve, Guff and Brunswick 2021). Combined with the higher risk of infection to front-line health workers, such developments could hollow out expertise and practitioner numbers for a generation, not only from attrition but by driving down recruitment.

One challenge of disinformation is that it not only encourages non-participation in mitigation measures and vaccination programs, but also motivates them to prevent others from doing so as well (Hunt 2020). In the roll-out of the vaccine in the US, protestors blocked mass vaccination sites, burned vaccination infrastructure, and threatened the healthcare workers who staff them (Kika 2021). In one incident a protestor rammed her car through an outdoor drive through COVID-testing site shouting "No Vaccine," endangering seven health care workers (Bella 2021). Security guards were hired to protect health workers "for the foreseeable future" at three mobile COVID vaccination sites in Colorado following harassment and vandalism including protestors throwing lit fireworks into the work site. One of the earliest and largest vaccination sites in the US was forced to shut down at Dodger Stadium in Los Angeles in January 2021 due to protestor blockades. The organizers, coordinating on social media, noted that "this is a march against everything COVID, Vaccine, PCR Tests, Lockdowns, Masks, Fauci, Gates, Newsom, China, digital tracking, etc," and in a nod to the political origins implored protestors to "please refrain from wearing Trump/MAGA attire as we want our statement to resonate with the sheeple" (Gerber and Khan 2021). These demonstrations are not limited to the United States. In Sydney, Australia a drive-through COVID testing site in Sydney's west was the target of an arson attack with the burned-out shell graffitied with "take back the power" and "COVID equals lies" (Riga 2021). It follows on from lockdown protests in Melbourne, Australia with protestors chanting "Arrest Bill Gates!"

The concomitant attack on research institutes and public health institutions such as the CDC, WHO and educational institutions, point to long-term problems of politicization and funding. Unfortunately, at a time when the population was most exposed to the twin viruses of the pandemic and conspiracy theories, the body politics' immune system was already being weakened. Erosion of trust in key institutions and professions such as scientific institutions, universities and the free press impacts the community's ability to respond to the pandemic with evidence-based policymaking. Public opinion polls have tracked Americans' gradual loss of trust in public institutions such as courts, law enforcement and legislative bodies. But the most disturbing trends have a partisan edge and are much more recent. A 2019 Pew report on higher education found that as of 2017, the majority of Republicans surveyed identified universities as a threat to the nation's well-being (Pew Research Centre 2019).

As the pandemic continued, the range of institutions under fire expanded from public health agencies to courts, school boards and local government. Town hall and school board meetings broadcast live have documented concerted efforts to undermine COVID-19 mitigation strategies such as masks and vaccines. Meanwhile public health officials and practitioners were threatened with violence. German virologist Christian Drosten received a parcel with a vial of liquid labelled "positive" and a letter telling him to drink it. In Belgium, a prominent virologist and his family were placed in a safe house when a military sniper broadcast his intentions to target virologists (Nogrady 2021). In Maryland, USA, a pharmacist was murdered for distributing the Covid-19 vaccine (Anderson 2021). These attacks have continued, expanding to key institutions accused of complicity or corruption during the pandemic. In February 2024, a US man beheaded his father for "being part of the Deep State" (he was a federal employee). He was later charged with terrorism, after authorities found bomb-making materials and plans for federal buildings (Catalini 2024). In this way, the allure of disinformation and conspiracy theories as a form of inside knowledge providing certainty and community in a time of great chaos makes them valuable political weapons ripe for violence. For instance, Qanon, a large online conspiracy theory community has leveraged concern about government malfeasance and child trafficking, to label COVID-19 a hoax and cover. These tactics were leveraged during the pandemic to drive extremist recruitment.

Driving Extremism

The weaponization of social media and the promulgation of extremist groups on Facebook has exacerbated challenges in nearly every policy area, from aiding terrorist recruitment, to being a state tool of great-power competition, to damaging the vitality of democracy (Singer and Brooking 2018). Before the pandemic, in mid-2019, an FBI memo warned against "conspiracy-driven domestic terrorism" (Winter 2019). One group identified in the report, QAnon, pivoted from its core message of child sex trafficking by political enemies (heir to the Pizzagate conspiracy theory) to COVID-related anti-government narratives. For instance, the QAnon #SaveTheChildren mantra was redirected to fight mitigation efforts in schools, including mask mandates and vaccination. When Facebook attempted to shut down Qanon groups, membership surpassed 1 million members across 15 countries. Even more concerning was the fact that 60% of membership arrives in the QAnon groups after Facebook's own group recommender directed them there (Wong 2020). Once arrived, it may not take long to radicalize the reader into acting on their newfound belief. For instance, convinced by the QAnon Pizzagate theory that a pizza parlor frequented by Democratic powerbrokers housed a basement for sex trafficking, a man from North Carolina travelled five hours to DC fully armed to "Save the Children." He instead terrorized a child's birthday party and served four years in prison. From the first time that he encountered the narrative online to loading up his vehicle with weapons for a five-hour drive, was a mere three days.

Allied nations reported a similar phenomenon. In Australia, the head of the Australian Secret Intelligence Organization (ASIO) warned in a rare public briefing that far-right extremists were exploiting coronavirus to gather new members. As reported by the *ABC*, "COVID-19 restrictions are being exploited by extreme right-wing narratives that paint the state as oppressive, and globalization and democracy as flawed and failing," the intelligence agency warned… "We assess the COVID-19 pandemic has reinforced an extreme right-wing belief in the inevitability of societal collapse and a 'race war'" (Christodoulou 2020). ASIO's Director General had earlier that year identified the far right as the fastest-growing extremist group in Australia: "In Australia, the extreme right-wing threat is real, and it is growing. In suburbs around Australia, small cells regularly meet to salute Nazi flags, inspect weapons, train in combat, and share their hateful ideology. These groups are more organized than they were in previous years" (ASIO Director General 2020).

The global reach of these groups is accelerated by technological connectivity and advancement in tools that automate and disseminate their message. Cyber-enabled disinformation has been the nexus of conspiracy-driven extremism. During COVID-19, conspiracy theories blaming technology, religious minorities, immigrants, secret cabals and political adversaries spread from the dark corners of the internet to Facebook group pages, to traditional media and public officials. These narratives implicitly rationalized violence. Narratives around 5G technology were coopted to rationalize destruction of critical infrastructure across the United Kingdom (UK), Australia and the Netherlands. According to Mobile UK, there were more than 90 arson attacks in the UK against mobile infrastructure, and more than 200 documented instances of abuse towards engineers in the first two months of the pandemic (Vincent 2020). According to the Asian Americans Advancing

Justice organization, which tracks hate crimes, more than 2,000 cases of assault were reported between March and June 2020, with perpetrators mirroring the rhetoric of "KungFlu" or "China virus" used by elected officials and influencers (Donaghue 2020).

Similar intimidation tactics targeted public health officials, state governors, scholars, researchers, philanthropists and other public figures on the front line of COVID-19 response. Later they would target local school boards and university leadership. These conspiracy theories helped to derail public health mitigation mandates as well as hinder vaccination efforts, and endangered scientific communities and educational practitioners. In an article entitled "I hope you die," a *Nature* survey of 300 scientists revealed the growing prevalence of threats against researchers in Germany, Australia and the US (Nogrady 2021). As extremist groups leverage disinformation to build their popularity to run for electoral office, they have come to directly influence policy-making and public funding.

Boosting Political Campaigns

The weakening of these scientific institutions and the fracturing of social trust provides opportunity for charlatans and conspiracy theorists to fill the vacuum, mounting their own electoral campaigns for power over decision-making and helping to oust office holders in their path. School board members reported intimidation and harassment efforts to force them from office. In Florida, a local school board member enacting COVID-19 measures described intimidation and credible threats of violence including armed men showing up at her home, being followed in her car, and bogus allegations to child protective services in an attempt to rob her of custody (Gallion 2021). In the same state, the governor DeSantis withheld pay from school board members who enacted masks mandates (Pedroja 2021). In their place, conspiracy-driven extremists are running for local, state and federal office to overturn mask mandates and vaccination efforts. Two Republican candidates backed by President Trump won high office in the 2020 election (and re-election again in 2022) on QAnon narratives, and consistently conflated mitigation efforts to Nazism. These include newly elected US Congresswoman Lauren Boebert (2021) tweeting that Biden "has deployed his Needle Nazis" and fellow Congresswomen Marjorie Taylor Green (R-GA) compared vaccination workers to "Nazi Brown shirts" and vaccine mandates as "segregation." During her electoral run, Marjorie Taylor Greene said of her candidacy against Democrats, "there's a once-in-a-lifetime opportunity to take this global cabal of Satan-worshiping pedophiles out" (Greene 2021). By smearing political opponents as pedophiles, Satanists, and Nazis, little cooperation or compromise is possible. This type of rhetoric undermines democratic functioning. These tactics trickled down to state-level government. A member of the Alaska legislature attempted to invoke the 1947 Nuremberg code to harass doctors who were distributing COVID-19 vaccines (Brooks 2021). In Kansas (August 2021), commissioners were confronted with an angry, mostly unmasked crowd before they mandated indoor public masks for 2- to-12-year-olds who are too young to be vaccinated. During four hours of public comment, opponents invoked the Holocaust, the Taliban, and Japanese internment camps (Kelleher et al. 2021). While stoked by hostile foreign actors, these narratives become more potent when picked up by domestic political actors, against which there are fewer avenues to address.

If we consider the global information commons akin to the natural environment, disinformation resembles pollution. Similar to twentieth-century pollution, a few main actors comprise the majority of the problem. A report from the Centre for Countering Digital Hate showed 12 anti-vaccine accounts spread nearly two-thirds of the anti-vaccine misinformation online (Center for Countering Digital Hate 2021). One of these "Disinformation Dozen," Robert F. Kenney Jr, who repeatedly invoked Nazis and the Holocaust when denouncing COVID-19 mitigation efforts, leveraged the pandemic to triple fundraising receipts for his anti-vaccine group, Children's Health Defense, and mounted a 2024 Presidential campaign (AP News 2023). However, the scale and the reach of a small number of actors cannot be underestimated. When a US celebrity tweeted an anecdote conflating STI symptoms with a COVID-19 vaccine response, the impacts were immediate and felt as far away as Trinidad and Tobago who publicly directed substantial resources to squashing the misinformation (Mendez 2021).

Meanwhile, large swathes of the global information ecosystem are privately owned. The financial motive of the platform owners to attract and hold users may at times compete with efforts to fight disinformation on their sites. A change in ownership can also drastically change moderation policies designed to combat foreign interference and disinformation campaigns. For instance, Twitter, while once lauded for its comprehensive moderation and safety protocols during COVID-19, saw a spike in disinformation regarding the pandemic after Elon Musk purchased the site and dismantled safety protocols. ABC News reported "Covid 19 and vaccine misinformation spiking on Twitter after Elon Mush fires moderators," (Purtill 2022) while researchers protested that API tools once freely distributed to detect and track disinformation were made inaccessible. Journalists, scientists and other health authorities also saw their reach on the site greatly diminished. As Politifact reported in 2023, "In the year since Elon Must purchased Twitter for $44 billion, the platform known as X has removed guardrails designed to restrict the flow of mis and disinformation, including stripping away what was once a free account verification process designed to combat impersonation, and replacing it with paid 'blue check' accounts that guarantee posts will be prioritized by X's algorithm" (Czopek 2023). Twitter, under Musk, also removed a key tool in the fight against disinformation warfare campaigns: labels that identified the origin of Russian, Chinese and Iranian state media accounts, which consequently surged 70% (NPR 2023). These changes demonstrate that global disinformation fighting tools embedded in private companies are potentially vulnerable to disruption.

Conclusion

Disinformation has significant and potentially long-lasting impacts. Over the last few years, cyber-enabled disinformation campaigns, both foreign and domestic, have altered what people read, share, believe and act upon. Trust in those who proffer facts – educational institutions, researchers, public health officials and health practitioners – has suffered a decline and undermined their influence. By eroding trust in scientific and government institutions and creating confusion over facts, disinformation stymes collective action and cooperation both domestically and with international partners. The Deputy Secretary of the North Atlantic Treaty Organization (NATO), Rose Gottemoeller (2018) called "alternative facts a threat to the alliance" as it undermines a sense of shared reality and a will to fight together against common challenges. The implications for national security are considerable. From climate to covid, disinformation hampers policy response.

In the competition for influence, the COVID-19 pandemic has demonstrated fruitful avenues to exploit by both hostile foreign powers and domestic partisans to reshape power and decision-making. As H. Colleen Sinclair argues, "Information warfare abounds and everyone online has been drafted- whether they know it or not" (Sinclair 2023). Democracies have steadily begun to bolster their collective defenses. Estonia, the target of one of earliest state-based cyber and information warfare attacks, has developed a model for education and civil cyber defense including information warfare. It has also collated international legal norms to address cyber-enabled disinformation campaigns, embodied in the *Tallin Manual 2.0* (see also NATO's International Cyber Law Interactive Toolkit 2021).

Stanford Professor of Cybersecurity, Herb Lin (2019) notes the difficulties of defense in securing the information global commons against disinformation threats – while traditional cybersecurity threats exploit the vulnerabilities of the system, these evolving attacks exploit its virtues, harnessing the openness and virality of social media. Countries like Finland have demonstrated that defenses are cross-disciplinary, in the social sciences and humanities. Finland has consistently topped the annual Media Literacy index measuring resistance to fake news and disinformation amongst 35 countries (Henley 2020; Media Literacy Index 2019). Social sciences research in psychology, political science and communication studies can also help support the design of counter-messaging strategies to fight disinformation. Meanwhile, governments that work closely with technology companies to identify extremist and illegal content such as Islamic State recruitment and child pornography rings, have turned their attention inward to fight conspiracy-driven domestic terrorism. New AI tools can assist, alongside a concerted effort in regulation, education and enforcement. For instance, while generative AI offers the potential to create disinformation narratives microtargeted at scale, the same technology can be used in crafting evidence-based messaging to suit different audiences to assist in countering public health misinformation, disinformation and conspiracy theories.

For the new future, however, health and emergency communication must compete with hostile foreign actors, profit seekers and snake oil salesmen for a valuable resource, attention. The implications of disinformation which undermines evidence-based discourse, decision-making and collective responses to crises will linger far after the pandemic itself. In the post-pandemic world, defense against this type of information warfare includes hardening targets through regulatory responses and educational campaigns. Social science provides insight into countering strategic narratives. Notably, when developers of the AstraZeneca vaccine, Gilbert and Greene decried the deleterious effects of disinformation, they agreed that, "certainly next time – and there will be a next time – we should include some political scientists on the team" (2021, 27). To survive the post-truth age, it is imperative that countries and allies strengthen their own capability and resilience in countering disinformation challenges to state stability in all its various forms.

Note

1 For example, see UK Foreign Office and Foreign and Commonwealth Office: Information Research Department: "Soviet disinformation operations" 1966 (FCO 168/2246); "Disinformation: note on Soviet aims and methods" 1967 (168/2843); "Disinformation activity by the KGB", 1970 (FCO168/4181), "disinformation: KGB Operational Methods 1970 (FCO 168/4188); UK Foreign Office and Foreign and Commonwealth Office: Northern Department and East European and Soviet Department, "Soviet Propaganda and Disinformation" 1983, (FCO 28/5813).

References

Anderson, J. (2021) "Maryland man allegedly fatally shot his pharmacist brother for 'killing people' with the COVID vaccine, court records show." *Baltimore Sun*, 7 October 2021. www.baltimoresun.com/news/crime/bs-md-cr-burnham-follow-20211006-srubyenoujenvkd5igalidruwm-story.html

ASIO Director General. (2020) "1st annual threat assessment." Speech delivered at Canberra, Australia, 4 February 2020. www.asio.gov.au/director-generals-annual-threat-assessment.html

Associated Press. (2023) "Anti-vaccine activist RFK Kr. launches presidential campaign." *AP News*, 11 April 2023. https://apnews.com/article/kennedy-biden-president-2024-democrat-dd9d6ecf17b54f4b32e7b17778540431

Auschwitz Museum. (2020) *Twitter @AuschwitzMuseum*, 2 May 2020. https://twitter.com/AuschwitzMuseum/status/1256446016510930945?s=20

Baker, S. and Walsh, M. (2024) "How memes transformed from pics of cute cats to health disinformation superspreaders." *The Conversation*, 13 February 2024. https://theconversation.com/how-memes-transformed-from-pics-of-cute-cats-to-health-disinformation-super-spreaders-221680

Bella, T. (2021) " 'No vaccine!': Woman arrested for allegedly driving through vaccination site, nearly hitting workers." *Washington Post*, 27 May 2021. www.washingtonpost.com/nation/2021/05/27/covid-vaccine-car-protest-tennessee/

Bittman, L. (1985) *The KGB and Soviet Disinformation: An Insider's View*. (Washington: Pergamon-Brasseys).

Boebert, L. (2021) *Twitter @laurenboebert*, 8 June 2021. https://twitter.com/laurenboebert/status/1413103995967746051

Broniatowski, D., Jamison, A., Qi, S., Al Kulaib, L., Chen, T., Benton, A., Quinn, S. and Dredze. M. (2018) "Weaponised health communication: Twitter bots and Russian trolls amplify the vaccine debate." *American Journal of Public Health* 108, no. 10 (October 2018): 1378–1384. https://doi.org/10.2105/AJPH.2018.304567

Brooks, J. (2021) "Alaska House rejects vote on Nuremberg code pushed by COVID vaccine skeptics." *Anchorage Daily News*, 14 September 2021. www.adn.com/politics/alaska-legislature/2021/09/12/alaska-house-rejects-vote-on-nuremberg-code-a-topic-cited-by-covid-vaccine-skeptics/

Brown University (2022) "New analysis shows vaccines could have prevented 318,000 lives." *Global Epidemics, Brown University School of Public Health*, 13 May 2022. https://globalepidemics.org/2022/05/13/new-analysis-shows-vaccines-could-have-prevented-318000-deaths/

Bruns, R., Hosangadi, D., Trotochaud, M., et al. (2021). COVID-19 Vaccine Misinformation and Disinformation Costs an Estimated $50 to $300 Million Each Day. Johns Hopkins Center for Health Security, Baltimore, MD.

Catalini, M. (2024) "Man charged with beheading father carried photos of federal buildings, bomb plans, DA says." *Associated Press News*, 16 February 2024. https://apnews.com/article/father-beheaded-video-mohn-decapitation-b6122b0f8f05b509b243c2064a16344f

Center for Countering Digital Hate (CCDH) (2021) "The Disinformation Dozen: The Sequel." July 2021. www.counterhate.com/disinfosequel

Christodoulou, M. (2020) "ASIO briefing warns that the far right is exploiting coronavirus to recruit new members." *ABC*, 12 June 2020. www.abc.net.au/news/2020-06-12/asio-briefing-warns-far-right-is-exploiting-coronavirus/12344472

Clifford, T. (2021) "Man sentenced to 6 years in plot to kidnap Michigan governor." *Reuters*, 26 August 2021. www.reuters.com/world/us/man-sentenced-6-years-plot-kidnap-michigan-governor-2021-08-25/

Condon, S. (2013) "Supreme Court strikes down section of Voting Rights Act." 25 June 2013. www.cbsnews.com/news/supreme-court-strikes-down-section-of-voting-rights-act/

Czopek, M. (2023) "How Elon must ditched Twitter's safeguards and primed X to spread misinformation." *PolitiFact*, 23 October 2023. www.politifact.com/article/2023/oct/23/how-elon-musk-ditched-twitters-safeguards-and-prim/

Donaghue, E. (2020) "2,120 hate incidents against Asian Americans reported during Coronavirus pandemic." *CBS News*, 2 July 2020. www.cbsnews.com/news/anti-asian-american-hate-incidents-up-racism/

Evans, R. and Novak, R. (1979) "Moscow: Dirty tricks and disinformation." *Washington Post*, 16 February 1979.

Ferreira Caceres, M., Sosa, J., Lawrence, J., Sestacovschi, C., Tidd-Johnson, A., Rasool, M., Kumar, V., Gadamidi, S., Pandav, K., Cuevas-Lou, C., Parrish, M., Rodriguez, I., and Fernandez, J (2022). The impact of misinformation on the COVID-19 pandemic. *AIMS Public Health* 9, no. 2 (January 2022): 262–277. https://doi.org/10.3934/publichealth.2022018

Gallion, B. (2021) "School Board member Jennifer Jenkins comments about threats, harassment grab national attention." *Florida Today*, 14 October 2021. www.floridatoday.com/story/news/education/2021/10/14/jennifer-jenkins-details-threats-harassment-over-mask-vote/8450501002/

Gerber, M. and Khan, I. (2021) "Dodger Stadium's COVID-19 vaccination site temporarily shut down after protesters gather at entrance." *Los Angeles Times*, 30 January 2021. www.latimes.com/california/story/2021-01-30/dodger-stadiums-covid-19-vaccination-site-shutdown-after-dozens-of-protesters-gather-at-entrance

Gilbert, S. and Green, C. (2021) *Vaxxers: The Inside Story of the Oxford AstraZeneca Vaccine and the Race Against the Vaccine* (London: Hodder and Soughton).

Gottemoeller, R. (2018) Shangri-la Security Dialogue, Singapore, 2 June 2018.

Green, M. T. (2021) *Twitter @mtgreenee Twitter*, 26 July 2021. https://twitter.com/mtgree nee/status/1419489724985643008

Henley, J. (2020) "How Finland starts its fight against fake news in primary schools." *The Guardian*, 29 January 2020. www.theguardian.com/world/2020/jan/28/fact-from-fiction-finlands-new-lessons-in-combating-fake-news

Hillis, S., Unwin, J., Che, Y., Cluver, L., Sherr, L., Goldman, P., Ratmann, O., Donnelly, C., Bhatt, S., Villaveces, A., Butchart, A., Bachman, G., Rawlings, L., Green, P., Nelson, C., and Flaxman S. "Global minimum estimates of children affected by COVID-19-associated orphanhood and deaths of caregivers: A modelling study." *The Lancet* 398, no. 10298 (July 2021): 391 – 402.

Hunt, J. (2020) "The COVID-19 pandemic v post truth." Global Health Security Network, Policy Report No. 1, 1 September 2020. www.ghsn.org/Policy-Reports

Hunt, J. (2021) "Countering cyber-enabled disinformation: Implications for national security" *Australian Journal of Defense and Strategic Studies* 3, no. 1 (July 2021): 83–88.

International Cyber Law interactive Toolkit, NATO Cooperative Cyber Defence Centre of Excellence, Tallin, Estonia (2021). https://cyberlaw.ccdcoe.org/wiki/Main_Page

Jack, C. (2017). *Lexicon of Lies: Terms for Problematic Information* (New York: Data and Society). https://datasociety.net/pubs/oh/DataAndSociety_LexiconofLies.pdf

Kelleher, J., Tang, T., Rodriguez, O. (2021) "Mask, vaccine conflicts descend into violence and harassment." *AP News*, 22nd August 2021. https://apnews.com/article/health-coro navirus-pandemic-2eba81ebe3bd54b3bcde890b8cf11c70

Kika, T. (2021) "Security guards to accompany mobile vaccination unites after harassment by anti-vaxxers." *Newsweek*, 11 September 2021. www.newsweek.com/security-guards-accompany-mobile-vaccination-units-after-harassment-anti-vaxxers-1628202

Lin, H. (2019) "Cyber operations v. information operations." *11th International Conference on Cyber Conflict (Cycon)*, Tallinn, Estonia, May 2019. www.youtube.com/watch?v= KyCDvEzq25s

Mendez, R. (2021) "UK and Trinidad health officials refute Nicki Minaj's false claim Covid shots cause swollen testicles." *CNBC*, 15 September 2021. www.cnbc.com/2021/09/15/ nicki-minaj-health-officials-in-uk-and-trinidad-refute-false-claim-covid-shots-cause-swollen-testicles-.html

Mitchell, A., Jurkowitz, M., Oliphant B., and Shearer, E. (2020) "Three months in, many Americans see exaggeration, conspiracy theories, partisanship in COVID-19 news." *Pew Research Center*, 29 June 2020. www.pewresearch.org/journalism/2020/06/29/ three-months-in-many-americans-see-exaggeration-conspiracy-theories-and-partisans hip-in-covid-19-news/

Mossburg, C., Waldrop, T., Thomas, N., (2020) "Public health officials are resigning amid threats during the COVID-19 pandemic." *CNN*, 23 June 2020.

Moye, D. (2021) "Pro-trump speaker wants to turn DC rally into 'mass-spreader event.'" *HuffPost*, 5 January 2021. www.huffpost.com/entry/clay-clark-trump-dc-rally-mass-spreader-event_n_5ff4e12cc5b6ec8ae0b69f57?ncid=tweetlnkushpmg00000067

NBC News (2021) "My dad didn't have a fighting chance: Covid is leading cause of death among law enforcement." *NBC News*, 17 September 2021. www.nbcnews.com/news/us-news/it-doesn-t-have-happen-covid-leading-cause-death-among-n1279289

Nogrady, B. (2021) "'I hope you die;' How the Covid pandemic unleased attacks against scientists." *Nature*, 14 October 2021. www.nature.com/articles/d41586-021-02741-x

NPR (2022) "Their mom died of COVID. They say conspiracy theories are what killed her." *All Things Considered Podcast*, 24 April 2022. www.npr.org/sections/health-shots/2022/ 04/24/1089786147/covid-conspiracy-theories

NPR (2023) "Twitter once muzzled Russian and Chinese state propaganda. That's over now." *All Things Considered Podcast*, 21 April 2023. www.npr.org/2023/04/21/1171193 551/twitter-once-muzzled-russian-and-chinese-state-propaganda-thats-over-now

O'Keefe, S. (2020) "One in three Americans would not get COVID 19 vaccine." Gallup online 7 August 2020. One in Three Americans Would Not Get COVID-19 Vaccine (gallup.com).

Pedroja, C. (2021) "Florida Gov. Ron DeSantis threatens to withhold pay of School Boards who require mask." *Newsweek*, 9 August 2021. www.msn.com/en-us/news/us/florida-gov-ron-desantis-threatens-to-withhold-pay-of-school-boards-who-require-masks/ar-AAN7K1F

Pew Research Center (2019) "The growing partisan divide in views of higher education." August 2019. www.pewresearch.org/social-trends/2019/08/19/the-growing-partisan-div ide-in-views-of-higher-education-2/

Purtill, J. "Covid-19, vaccine misinformation spiking on Twitter after Elon Musk fires moderators." *ABC News*, 8 December 2022. www.abc.net.au/news/science/2022-12-08/ covid-misinformation-spiking-on-twitter-elon-musk/101742276

Reeve, E., Guff, S., and Brunswick, D. (2021) "The surreal lives of Arkansas nurses fighting Covid-19 inside the hospital and denial on the outside." *CNN*, 23 July 2021. https://edit ion.cnn.com/2021/07/22/us/arkansas-covid-nurse-vaccine/index.html

Richardson, R. (2020) "From cold to cannibalism: Rush Limabugh's whiplash inducing evolution on the Covid pandemic." *Mediaite*, 15 July 2020.

Rid, T. (2020) *Active Measures: The Secret History of Disinformation and Political Warfare* (London: Profile Books).

Riga, J. (2021) "Drive through test site was Sydney's west target of possible arson attack." *ABC News Blog*, 29 August 2021 www.abc.net.au/news/2021-08-29/covid-live-blog-nsw-press-conference-vic-lockdown/100415572

Saletan, W. (2020) "The trump pandemic." *Slate*, 9 August 2020. https://slate.com/news-and-politics/2020/08/trump-coronavirus-deaths-timeline.html.

Shane, L. (2019) "Overseas trolls targeting veterans on social media: Report." *Military Times*, 18 September 2019. www.militarytimes.com/news/pentagon-congress/2019/09/ 17/overseas-trolls-targeting-veterans-on-social-media-report/

Sinclair, H. C. (2023) "Disinformation is rampant on social media: A social psychologist explains the tactics used against you." *The Conversation*, 8 December 2023. https://thec onversation.com/disinformation-is-rampant-on-social-media-a-social-psychologist-expla ins-the-tactics-used-against-you-216598

Singer, P. W. and Brooking, E. T. (2018). *Like War: The Weaponization of Social Media* (Boston: Mariner Books).

Starbird, K., Arif, A., and Wilson, T. (2019) "Disinformation as collaborative work: Surfacing the participatory nature of strategic information operations." *Proceedings of the ACM on Human Centred Interaction*. https://faculty.washington.edu/kstarbi/StarbirdArifWilson_ DisinformationasCollaborativeWork-CameraReady-Preprint.pdf

Swift, J. (1710) "Political lying." *The Examiner*, 1710. www.bartleby.com/lit-hub/english-prose-an-anthology-in-five-volumes/jonathan-swift-16671745-18/

Trump, D. (2020) "Liberate Michigan." *Twitter @RealDonaldTrump*, 17 April 2020. https:// twitter.com/realDonaldTrump/status/1251169217531056130

UK Foreign Office and Foreign and Commonwealth Office (1966) Information Research Department: "Soviet disinformation operations." 1966 (FCO 168/2246), London Archives, Accessed 10 October 2022.

US Director of National Intelligence (DNI) (2017) "Assessing Russian activities and intentions in recent US elections." US Intelligence Community Assessment, ICA 2017-01D, 6 January 2017.

US Senate Intelligence Report on Russian Interference in the 2016 Election Vol 1–5 (2019). Washington DC. www.intelligence.senate.gov/publications/report-select-committee-intel ligence-united-states-senate-russian-active-measures

US State Department (2020) GEC Special Report: Russia's Pillars of Disinformation and Propaganda. Washington DC, August 2020. www.state.gov/wp-content/uploads/ 2020/08/Pillars-of-Russia%E2%80%99s-Disinformation-and-Propaganda-Ecosystem_ 08-04-20.pdf

Vincent, J. (2020) "Something in the air – Conspiracy theorists say 5G causes novel coronavirus, so now they're attacking UK telecoms engineers." *The Verge*, 3 June 2020. www.theverge.com/2020/6/3/21276912/5g-conspiracy-theories-coronavirus-uk-telec oms-engineers-attacks-abuse

Watts, C. (2017) Testimony to US Senate Intelligence Committee. Washington DC, 30 March 2017. www.intelligence.senate.gov/sites/default/files/documents/os-cwatts-033 017.pdf .

Wilson, J. (2021) "'Tyranny': US rightwingers portray nightmare vision of Australia's covid response." *The Guardian*, 10 October 2021. www.theguardian.com/australia-news/2021/ oct/10/tyranny-us-rightwingers-portray-nightmare-vision-of-australias-covid-response

Winter, J. (2019) "Exclusive: FBI document warns conspiracy theories are a new domestic terrorism threat." *Yahoo News*, 2 August 2019. https://news.yahoo.com/fbi-documents-conspiracy-theories-terrorism-160000507.html

Wong, J. (2020) "Revealed QAnon Facebook Groups are growing at a rapid pace around the world." *The Guardian*, 11 August 2020. www.theguardian.com/us-news/2020/aug/11/ qanon-facebook-groups-growing-conspiracy-theory

World Economic Forum (2024) Global Risks Report, 10 January 2024. www.weforum.org/ publications/global-risks-report-2024/

World Health Organisation (2020) "Attacks on health care in the context of COVID-19." 30 July 2020. www.who.int/news-room/feature-stories/detail/attacks-on-health-care-in-the-context-of-covid-19

Yablokov, I. (2015) "Conspiracy theories as a Russian public diplomacy tool: The case of *Russia Today (RT)*." *Politics* 35, no. 3 (April 2015): 301–315. https://doi.org/10.1111/ 1467-9256.12097

Part III

Improving Health Security Threat and Risk Mitigation

5 Building Better Health Security Intelligence Strategies Post-COVID-19

Gemma Bowsher

Introduction

COVID-19 has marked a period of substantial rupture in international norms across both the security and global health fields. The pandemic has been described as 'the 9/11 of health security' (Daoudi 2020), signalling its profound impact on reordering security priorities at national and international scales. Global health security (GHS) approaches have been consolidated across international health regimes, driven by organisations such as the World Health Organization (WHO) and national governments. Emerging innovations in financing, intelligence and preparedness are building upon pandemic failures, placing health security approaches at the centre of reform and recovery efforts (White House 2022).

Reflection on weaknesses in international COVID-19 responses repeatedly raise the issue of intelligence as a critical failure across governance, health and security fields (IPPPR 2021; Bowsher & Sullivan 2021). International collaboration in this regard has been notable for its lack of strategic awareness on the emerging threat of SARS-CoV-2. Additionally, intelligence alliances, such as 'Five Eyes' have been challenged to counter a range of unique threats both within and well beyond their traditional remits. Furthermore, diverse political approaches to disease responses have polarised the advancement of common goals and revealed a health security machinery that poorly integrates intelligence approaches across the 'Five Eyes' alliance and beyond (Bowsher et al. 2020).

The complexity of the biosphere[1] presents novel intelligence requirements cutting across existing geo-political tectonics. Biological risks extend the traditional remit of 'Five Eyes'. Under the health security framing, issues such as climate change, ecological destruction and wildlife extinction intersect with information warfare, territorial disputes and cyber hostilities to produce a threat paradigm requiring expanding interdisciplinary attention. Zoonotic diseases (pathogens transmitted between animal and human populations) such as SARS-CoV-2, Ebola and MERS have demonstrated the volatility of this space as well as the lack of durable international infrastructure for combatting pandemic threats.

The pandemic has also driven an unprecedented convergence of information production around a singular threat entity to produce an expanding platform of intelligence approaches for use in both the national and security and public health

DOI: 10.4324/9781003335511-8

contexts (West et al. 2021; 89–102). Organisations from sectors across health, security and civil governance have reconfigured their operations to generate intelligence to detect and respond to the multivalent, pan-societal disruption of the pandemic (Davis 2020). In addition, the evolution of technologies from genomic sequencing to big data has altered technical and organisational approaches to the production of intelligence as well as shifting overriding strategic priorities for future agendas (Bernard, Bowsher & Sullivan 2020, Shapira 2020). The ascendance of open-source intelligence (OSINT) has further drawn national intelligence agencies out of the shadows into a diverse ecosystem of intelligence providers (Janeva et al. 2022).

COVID-19 has also exposed the centrality of information as a prime currency for health security action across sectors and geographies. With informational approaches such as surveillance being expanded globally, intelligence approaches at the national and international level are becoming a lever around which information is increasingly transformed into policy action. This need to deliver information on the spreading pandemic, and its wider effects has galvanised diverse intelligence communities in the public and private sectors that have been operating within, and at the boundaries of health security risks over many decades (Walsh 2020; Walton 2020).

This chapter examines recent 'Five Eyes' political and operational planning emerging from the governments of these countries and explores how articulations of health security intelligence could be further established within national and international strategies. It asks how the machinery of 'Five Eyes' security, public health and intelligence sectors can be organised to deliver improved integrated domestic and international responses to health security emergencies. Finally, it explores how 'Five Eyes' can better rationalise its strategic commitments to health security, whilst continuing to address the full diversity of global threats from cyberwarfare, to conflict and terrorism.

Where Have We Reached with Health Security Intelligence?

Accompanying the growth of intelligence practice in response to health security threats, there are a broad spectrum of associated themes, methods and tools (Lentzos & Goodman 2020). No singular definition of health security intelligence exists that clarifies the discipline's boundaries based on its observed practices both before and during COVID-19 (Walsh 2020b). Disease surveillance and the mitigation of biological weapons lie at the heart of the earliest explicit approaches to the use of intelligence practices to inform health and biological strategies. As the Global Health Security (GHS) movement has coalesced, the centrality of surveillance has grown and complexified in line with emerging technologies (Lakoff 2018).

The security sector has become more overt in its role as an intelligence actor working in health security. In particular, the 'Five Eyes' Alliance has demonstrated novel commitments to health security collaboration. The countries of the alliance – the United Kingdom, the United States of America, Canada, Australia and New Zealand – have each employed unique approaches to the pandemic (UK Gov 2020, Pfluke 2019). 'Five Eyes' nations have delivered a range of pandemic-associated intelligence programmes from countering disinformation, to supporting medical capability assessments (Wilson et al. 2022). Public announcements from various intelligence agencies have demonstrated a greater willingness to deliver public intelligence products in the health security field particularly in the cyber and influence-associated domains (CSE 2020, Sengupta 2020). In January 2023 the US Director of National Intelligence took the rare step of declassifying the National Intelligence Estimate examining the 'Economics and National Security Implications of the COVID-19 Pandemic through 2026', once again signalling increasing efforts at transparency in the health security domain from Five Eyes Intelligence agencies (NIC 2022).

The establishment of the WHO Hub for Pandemic and Epidemic Intelligence is emblematic of parallel strategic shifts by non-governmental health actors to prioritising intelligence-based approaches to improving epidemiological data. The unit's mission to 'detect new events with pandemic potential and to monitor disease control measures on a real-time basis' represents the acknowledgement of intelligence as a relevant form of praxis within the international health security apparatus. This increasing receptivity towards intelligence approaches in organisations such as the WHO, and the newly instituted US CDC Centre for Forecasting and Outbreak and Analytics, signals the scope to enhance existing epidemiological intelligence with lessons from national security early warning principles. The G7 intergovernmental forum expressed its support for these approaches at the 2021 Carbis Bay Summit where it commissioned a One Health Intelligence Review (G7 2021). The United Kingdom's Integrated Review of Security, Defence, Development and Foreign Policy in 2021 has declared the UK Government commitment to strengthening 'analytical, policy and operational tools – including the collection and use of data – to better assess cross-cutting, complex risks' including health (Cabinet Office 2021, G7 2021). The Review also announced that the UK 'will adopt a new approach to preparedness and response to risks, which fully recognises that natural hazards and other risks can cause as much disruption to the UK's core interests as security threats' (Cabinet Office 2021; 87). Such pronouncements cement shifts in security policy, placing intelligence collection on natural hazards squarely within national security matrices, and expanding the bounds of governance action in this domain. This is further bolstered by the Review's acknowledgement that 'we have increased our Five Eyes cooperation, including in response to the pandemic, and will seek to strengthen policy cooperation further on a range of issues' (ibid). The 'Five Eyes' intelligence partnership has not previously declared involvement in health security working, and this represents an important acknowledgement of the impetus provided by the pandemic to re-orient security doctrines and bring to bear traditional security sector intelligence approaches to evolving pandemic threats.

Intelligence Communities Convene Around COVID-19

By the time of the first official notice of an outbreak of atypical pneumonia in Wuhan on 31 December 2019, reports had been circulating for several weeks amongst intelligence communities that an outbreak was unfolding in the city (Markson 2021, Wilson 2022). In March 2020, the leaders of the G7 released a statement stressing the value of 'real-time information sharing to ensure access to the best and latest intelligence, improving prevention strategies and mitigation measures… we will pool epidemiologic and other data to better understand and fight the virus' (G7 2020).

Subsequently, COVID-19 has drawn diverse security and intelligence communities together around a singular threat entity to reveal the potential of a biological phenomenon – a pandemic – to disrupt 'business as usual' through a complex web of health, security and wider social effects (Bricknell & Horne 2020). Early critiques of pandemic response have centred on the 'failure' of intelligence communities to identify and action early warning signals (Omand 2020; Levy & Wark 2021; Briggs et al. 2022; Bronskill 2020; Dahl 2023). The Canadian Global Public Health Intelligence Network (GPHIN) was deemed by an Independent Review Panel, not to be 'operating as clearly or smoothly as it should' (PHAC 2021). The panel raised the important point that for 'GPHIN to succeed, it must be situated within an environment that makes the best use of the intelligence it produces', with particular attention required towards connection with risk assessment functions (ibid.).

The close alignment of intelligence and health communities called for in various national defence and biosecurity strategies (e.g. UK, US and Canadian) was deemed inadequate in providing early notice and threat assessment (Zenko 2020). Intelligence communities have, however, been integral to the response phase of the pandemic, reflecting a shared threat mission across varying approaches and cultures (Shapira 2020). Epidemic intelligence organisations have been at the forefront of outbreak surveillance – spanning national and international organisations such as the UK Health Security Agency (UKHSA), GPHIN, CDC, WHO and European Union (Baker et al. 2021). These activities have included the monitoring of disease signal via tools such as indicator-based surveillance, genomic surveillance and increasingly open-source intelligence through event-based surveillance tools.

National security communities and their intelligence infrastructure have also been tasked with pandemic-related functions ranging from medical capacity and capability assessments, for example monitoring and sourcing PPE, to assessing potential concealed outbreaks in 'rogue' states such as North Korea (Migliore et al. 2021; Wilson et al. 2022). Domestically, both the Australian Criminal Intelligence Commission and the US NCMI were involved in public health functions such as contact tracing, disease modelling and logistics support (Walsh 2020; Walton 2020).

The second order effects of COVID-19 have also been clear targets of 'Five Eyes intelligence organisations. Alongside the direct health consequences of the virus, hostile nation states, criminal and extremist groups have been emboldened by shifts in national and international orders precipitated by pandemic disruption (Babb & Wilner 2021). Weaponisation of the information environment has been a notable phenomenon of the coronavirus experience (see Chapter 4). When the Director General of the WHO, Tedros Adhanom Ghebreyesus announced that the world was fighting both a pandemic and an 'infodemic', it signalled the growing impact of the cyber risks in health security (Zarocostas 2020). Intelligence organisations worldwide were tasked with tackling these issues; the UK announced that its signals intelligence (SIGINT) organisation, GCHQ and the British military intelligence organisation 77 Brigade were working on COVID-19 disinformation from hostile nation states, as well as supporting cyber-security functions of vaccine development and healthcare sector entities (Sengupta 2020, Young 2020). Similar responses were seen across 'Five Eyes' allies (Wark 2020, Walsh 2020a), Whether through exploitation of digitally dependent systems through cyber-attacks or via the spread of mis- and disinformation, information warfare ascended as a critical 'extra-viral' dimension of the COVID-19 threat (Bernard et al. 2020).

Building Better Health Security Intelligence Post-COVID-19

COVID-19 emerged amidst an already challenging international security environment. Intelligence agencies across 'Five Eyes' were occupied with the demands of countering foreign interference, cyber warfare and deteriorating regional security in critical areas such as the Indo-Pacific and Europe, when the pandemic emerged to provide a further fulcrum for hostility and insecurity. Unsurprisingly, despite key synergies between national security intelligence communities and the associated threats of a health security emergency, they had not sought to invest in what Walsh (2020a) has described as 'bureaucratic bandwidth' into making disease outbreaks a national intelligence priority.

This operational reality sits in contrast with the longstanding acceptance at the top tier of policy-making that disease outbreaks occupy a conceptual space in the same territory as regular national security threats. Professor Sir David Omand, the former director of GCHQ, has written: 'During my time as UK Intelligence and Security Coordinator after 9/11, a mutated flu pandemic occupied the top right-hand corner of the strategic notice risk matrix — of all the threats and risks, it poses the most lethal potential combination of impact and probability' (Omand 2020). Despite this recognition, the responses to COVID-19 demonstrated the effects of several decades of inadequate biodefence strategies across Five Eyes nations, with insufficient attention directed towards integrated inter-agency and international approaches to emerging biological threats.

Now that 'Five Eyes' has confirmed its involvement in various facets of the COVID-19 response, it is valuable to reflect on how a coherent programme of local and global operations can be maintained to support evolving health security intelligence platforms. Delivering improved health security intelligence is an attainable goal of 'Five Eyes' allies; strengths across a range of complex intersecting threat paradigms mark a high capability alliance in need of a concrete operational plan to ensure future success (Bowsher 2021).

Command and Control

The first challenge to such a programme of work centres upon the disparate nature of health security intelligence production and its connection to decision-makers across the nations of 'Five Eyes'. The responsibility for dealing with infectious disease threats such as COVID-19 tends to lie across a range of national and sub-national health authorities with varying involvement of national security intelligence organisations. In practice, this resulted in a dearth of organisations generating focused health security intelligence, with limited cohesion across domains to orient collection processes within an overarching threat paradigm.

During COVID-19, one of the first domestic developments across some 'Five Eyes' states was to stand up their respective advisory bodies composed of subject matter experts to inform high-level decision-making processes. In the UK, this took the form of the Scientific Advisory Group for Emergencies (SAGE), chaired by the Chief Scientific Advisor, in Australia the Health Protection Principal Committee drew together state and territory Chief Medical Officers, and the US stood up the 'White House Coronavirus Taskforce' (Jarman et al. 2022; Freedman 2020). Feeding into these committees were various sub-committees, health, security and intelligence authorities, with the final responsibility for decision-making lying with political leaders. These entities represented an attempt to coordinate diverse pools of information into a coherent platform for decision-making in the health security space. Nevertheless, criticisms cited issues with accountability, transparency, and the translation of evidence into advisory outputs and consequently, decisions taken by political leaders. Although leaders regularly cited their intention to 'follow the science', the mechanisms through which emerging evidence were parsed through structured information management processes to support political decisions were relatively variable and opaque (Vickery et al. 2022).

Such criticisms have been explored in emerging literatures spanning intelligence studies and sociological analyses of COVID-19 governance. The Science and Technology Studies (STS) scholars Collins and Evans (2002) have previously sought to delineate the boundaries between the 'scientific' and the 'political' by considering the differences between political and technical phases of decision-making processes, even when both are underpinned by the insights of best available (and often incomplete) scientific evidence. Robert Evans (2022) has argued that a key distinction of these elements lies in what participants are trying to achieve; the 'technical' being 'to act scientifically' and the 'political', to 'act in accordance with democratic principles'. Evans and other scholars (including the author) have questioned whether bodies such as SAGE and the White House taskforce were tasked with appropriate questions, or intelligence requirements by policymakers (Evans 2022; Bowsher & Sullivan 2021a). Common pathways of evidence uptake and expression of uncertainty are integral within intelligence frameworks, however a key criticism of political leadership across several poorly performing 'Five Eyes' nations has been the political reliance on scientific discourse with limited open acknowledgement of uncertainty within the technical advice provided. Documentation from SAGE and other advisory bodies did convey this uncertainty, however political messaging that characterising 'the science' as deterministic of policy production obfuscated some of the more contentious elements of pandemic governance during the emergency response phase (Freedman 2020). Subsequent recognition by Governments such as the Biden Administration of the uncertainty regarding COVID-19 origins, as expressed in the declassified NIE, has begun to open up discussions of the challenge of science-policy translation during health emergencies.

The translation of data into actionable products for policymaking audiences is a central objective of intelligence processes. Both the procedural and conceptual distinction between 'science' and 'intelligence' is important when considering the necessity of high stakes decision-making; the author has outlined the role of the intelligence cycle and its application to complex bio-emergencies which, as in other scientifically-informed security-relevant domains, bridge sometimes contentious divides between technical and political communities (Bowsher et al. 2020, Bowsher & Sullivan 2021a). At its simplest, this approach requires the operationalisation of the intelligence cycle in health security information management across governmental networks. The structured process beginning with 'direction' moving through 'collection, analysis, production and dissemination' ensures at a minimum, a common pathway of information processing in a multi-source, data-rich ecosystem (ibid). Essential dimensions of this undertaking include the response to specific, and appropriate intelligence requirements, as well as deploying the appropriate form of intelligence collection strategy to the requirement at hand. Subsequent analysis demands key expert stakeholders and inter-thematic liaison to appropriately weight the risks, costs and uncertainties. Finally generating tailored intelligence products appropriate to audience is vital to ensure impact upon dissemination to support the separate role of decision-makers. Calls for the clearer adoption of such an approach were made early in the pandemic by experts such as the former Secretary of the US Department of Homeland Security, Michael Chertoff, who proposed the creation of a Global Corona Intelligence Analysis Center (GCIAC) to pool international information and even 'help track the potential for rogue states and terrorists to weaponise pandemics' (Chertoff et al. 2020).

Clarity in these processes provides important accountability and transparency for government work, even when the content of intelligence products and process of deliberations require a degree of sensitivity and even secrecy. Constructing an effective operational-policy apparatus both within and between 'Five Eyes' states is crucial to delivering a rational approach to health security intelligence across the alliance. The revised 2023 UK Biosecurity Strategy has laid out a much clearer framework for this purpose, which clarifies roles and taskings and outlines the overriding strategic enablers to support integrated workflows (HM Gov 2023). Relationships between intelligence functions such as those within the Cabinet Office, the Ministry of Defence (MOD), and other security-oriented functions are mapped in relation to the UK Health Security Agency (UKHSA), Foreign Commonwealth and Development Office (FCDO) and other government departments. This evolution reflects institutional recognition of failures in integration and inter-operational working of intelligence and capabilities during COVID-19, and maximises the varied functions within the UK health security apparatus.

There are various infrastructure-based means with which to integrate a greater 'intelligence mindset' for health security within 'Five Eyes' nations. National intelligence communities have already shown the value of the intelligence fusion centres which classically work across inter-sectoral thematic fields on a range of issues such as terrorism and cyber. Across 'Five Eyes', fusion centres such as the Canadian Integrated Terrorism Assessment Centre, the UK Joint Terrorism Assessment Centre, the Australia National Threat Assessment Centre, the New Zealand Combined Threat Assessment Group and the US National Counterterrorism Center have proven the role for national foci that collate, integrate and analyse data from across member organisations and then disseminate intelligence products to relevant government departments. Domains such as health security, which encompass broad information from a wide array of sources are good candidates for intelligence fusion organisations.

The UK has taken up this approach through institutional reform of its health security infrastructure. In May 2020 the Joint Biosecurity Centre (JBC) was established to bring together data science, assessment and public health expertise on COVID-19 to support regional and local health leaders. This unit and national public health governance bodies (Public Health England) have subsequently been consolidated under the auspices of the newly established UK Health Security Agency (UKHSA), now responsible for 'protecting every member of every community from the impact of infectious diseases, chemical, biological, radiological and nuclear incidents and other health threats' (UKHSA 2024). Its mandate reaches further to connect 'scientific and operational leadership at national and local level, as well as on the global stage, to make the nation's health secure'. The UKHSA is an important exemplar of a form of health security organisation housing fusion capabilities (albeit with an extended remit as the designated national public health agency), which is focused on a theme, tasked with handling diverse forms of information – e.g. genomic surveillance, population indicators, clinical data and sensitive biological research data – and provided with a mandate for producing and sharing health security intelligence regionally or by geographic need.

Calls for a greater adoption of health security intelligence fusion approaches across 'Five Eyes' build on arguments that the ability of states to neutralise biological threats depends on their 'aggressive and pre-emptive response'. Scholars such as Albert et al. (2023) have suggested that the US establishes at least one 'epi-intel' fusion centre within each State, with a structured staffing roster encompassing key agencies to support the effective passage of intelligence from the States to the Federal government and vice versa. Canadian mechanisms for information sharing may centre on reviving and revitalising the health security function of the ITAC and institutionalising greater connection across the Public Health Agency of Canada (PHAC) and devolved provincial agencies. Further Canadian evolutions have included the creation of the Canadian Centre for Integrated Risk Assessment (CIRA) which operates under an all-hazards plan that 'defines the framework within which the Public Health Agency of Canada (PHAC) and Health Canada (HC) will operate to ensure an appropriate response to any emergency' (PHAC 2023). Of course, fusion is one way to organise intelligence functions, and may be an appropriate goal in the context of health security intelligence involving multiple disparate data sources and agencies. Fusion approaches however, have not been without criticism in other national security contexts, such as policing, with the central lesson emerging that there is no 'quick fix' to complex 'analytical issues of mutual concern' involving varied actors, organisations and interests (Walsh 2014).

Intra'-Five Eyes' cooperation can be consolidated in the health security space through the established information sharing and liaison networks already adopted across the alliance on other key security themes. 'Five Eyes' Intelligence sharing can take many forms, involving co-located liaison networks, multi-actor locations, fusion networks and common access databases/servers (Pfeifer 2012; Bowsher 2021). Medical intelligence is already shared through mechanisms such as the Quadripartite Medical Intelligence Committee involving the US, UK, Canada and Australia. Sharing can also be informal and ad hoc, without formal partnership mechanisms in place, but actioned on a 'need to know' basis if delivering time critical information of value to actors in relation to specific threats. There is scope for the creation of a cadre of 'health security liaison officers' to disseminate expertise across the intelligence agencies of the alliance in the same manner as is done for signals intelligence (SIGINT). The recent announcement by the US Secretary of State Anthony Blinken of plans for establishing a Bureau of Global Health Security and Diplomacy represents an opportunity for locating liaison-foci across similar 'Five Eyes' national bodies. Building on pre-pandemic commitments to use intelligence processes and collaborate with intelligence communities on health security matters would represent an import commitment across 'Five Eyes' to adopt more rational processes for evidence uptake and translation (HoC 2018).

Intelligence and Early Warnings

How the early signal of an emerging disease outbreak is detected is a challenging intelligence problem (Levy & Wark 2021; Wilson & McNamara 2020). Common and emerging pathogens appearing sporadically across large geographies pose enormous difficulties for international detection and surveillance systems (Bernard & Sullivan 2020). Intelligence communities have long grappled with how best to accommodate this widening spectrum of risks into a coherent operational strategy. It follows that to effectively monitor and forewarn of spreading risks, a degree of international cooperation and intelligence sharing is required across states, non-governmental networks, and increasingly private sector organisations. The sharing of early warning signal remains a key intelligence priority across 'Five Eyes' – media reports that signals of SARS-CoV-2 were shared across the Quadripartite alliance provide precedent for inter-allied sharing of outbreak early warnings (Brewster 2021). The field of early warnings however remains disparate, posing technical and regulatory challenges for the alliance. The key challenges for addressing many of the technical challenges in providing better early warning are discussed by Skillicorn in Chapter 6.

International surveillance networks such as Global Public Health Intelligence Network (GPHIN) and the Global Outbreak Alert and Response Network (GOARN) already operate as forms of open-source intelligence sharing across constituent member states. So too do certain mechanisms within the WHO's new Pandemic

Intelligence Hub such as the Epidemic Intelligence from Open Sources Initiative (EIOS). The growth of Open-Source Intelligence (OSINT) and other innovations such as artificial intelligence have upended traditional security sector activities by national intelligence agencies who have been forced to marry their existing capabilities with emerging technologies (Zegart 2023). Health security intelligence has experienced a strong drive to incorporate these tools also (Bernard et al. 2018). The abundance of forecasting and early warning tools in the private sector has produced an array of commercial entities such as *Blue Dot*, *Palantir* and *Metabiota* (Niiler 2020), which have supported early warning systems and response in settings such as the US, UK and Taiwan (Allam 2020). The Data science lead of *Metabiota* has reported that the company is working with the US intelligence agencies on COVID-19 issues as part of Metabiota's work with In-Q-Tel, a nonprofit venture associated with the CIA (Heilweil 2020). The Chinese company Hikivision has been used to provide facial recognition tools for COVID-19 positive individuals in European Commission buildings, and in 30 London Councils (Manancourt & Scott 2021).

Private sector involvement in support of national security intelligence functions is not a new phenomenon, however ethical concerns arise as the reliance on these organisations and their sometimes-opaque technologies escalates during health emergencies. Privacy concerns over the collection of population surveillance data by private entities warrant serious engagement by governments. Bernard et al. (2021a) have written of the expansion of bio-surveillance during the pandemic and the historical precedent for governments to retain such tools beyond the life cycle of a public health emergency (Davis 2021). A common operating framework for 'Five Eyes' States contracting out elements of health security intelligence infrastructure is warranted, in the same way that controls on foreign companies engaged with 'Five Eyes' digital infrastructure (e.g. Huawei) have previously been effected. Agreements such as the 2020 UK–US Agreement on Artificial Intelligence lays the foundation for coordinated bilateral research and development to cement intra-'Five Eyes' power bases, a theme that was subject to discussion during the November 2021 Annual Meeting of the Five Eyes Intelligence Oversight and Review Council (FIORC) (DNI 2021; UK Gov 2020).

Strengthening 'Intra-Five Eyes' clarity on the abundance of early warning tools and role for intelligence sharing in this space is a core goal if the alliance is to engage substantively on Health Security Intelligence. Further criticisms may be levelled that this abundance is part of the problem, and too many tools are not fit for purpose. Nevertheless, capability mapping and the conduction of robust validation assessments of emerging tools and platforms is a priority in a rapidly expanding, poorly regulated, multi-actor domain. Leadership through the form of formal multilateral agreements on outbreak early warning, or via expressions of support by political leaders for existing multilateral architectures such as the International Health Regulations and Pandemic Treaty negotiations, can articulate a commitment to longer-term support of health security objectives, including innovations in health security intelligence.

Evolving Geopolitics

The Russian invasion of Ukraine and the growing threat of China in the Indo-Pacific reiterate the enduring importance of 'Five Eyes' as a vital forum for cooperation around shared principles and pressing security threats. Hemmings and Varnish (2021) have cited the 'fluid informality' of the partnership which is maintained through shared values and common institutional approaches. This fluidity can also deliver agile and imaginative approaches to new and emerging intelligence priorities. Although the health security intelligence priority was firmly on the agendas of constituent nations, during the COVID-19 emergency, the challenge now will be how best to maintain this attention amidst an increasingly tumultuous geopolitical terrain.

The period since the onset of the COVID-19 pandemic has been beset by geopolitical turmoil and geostrategic realignments. The invasion of Ukraine, the escalation of Chinese hostilities in the Indo-Pacific and the continuing violence in regions such as the Sahel have placed health security in a complexifying field of overlapping security interests. The UK's Integrated Review and the US Security Strategy both cited the importance of Indo-pacific influence and the establishment of the AUKUS Pact between three of the Five Eyes nations – Australia, the US and the UK – signals these geostrategic shifts, in particular by articulating the role of Australia in asserting the 'Five Eyes' power base in the region. Further discussions are ongoing regarding the possible future inclusion of Japan in a 'Five Eyes +' alliance to bolster against growing regional Chinese influence (Walsh 2023).

Considering this trend in the context of health security intelligence, a number of geostrategic priorities emerge. The Indo-Pacific has long been held up as vulnerable to emerging outbreaks due to a combination of urban connectivity, expanding agriculture and an extensive animal trade. Concerns that major health security actors such as China have concealed emerging pandemics such as SARS-1 and SARS-CoV-2 have pushed states and multilateral organisations such as the World Health Organisation (WHO) to bolster regional disease surveillance infrastructure. The Indo Pacific has become a focus of Australian-led health security efforts through its Indo Pacific Centre for Health Security whose objective is to *'contribute to the avoidance and containment of infectious disease threats with the potential to cause social and economic harms on a national, regional or global scale'* (Australian Government 2019). The Centre possesses a range of functions including a Government Reference Group into which are seconded officials from a range of Australian Government Agencies. The Centre delivers vital situational awareness on a critical region of health security consequence. Other Indo Pacific health security programmes supported by 'Five Eyes members include cooperation between the Canadian Weapons Threat Reduction Programme (WTRP) and the ASEAN Emergency Operations Centre Network for public health emergencies that coordinates regional health security intelligence sharing with member states. Both of these mechanisms can be considered additional useful assets to 'Five Eyes' nations (ASEAN 2021).

Beyond the technical interventions, initiatives such as these leverage influence through health security diplomacy. The Indonesian granting of emergency use approval to a Chinese mRNA COVID-19 vaccine and Russian collaboration with the Brazilian Government on its Sputnik V Vaccine highlight the intraregional contestations being played out through COVID-19 diplomacy (Reuters 2022). Leveraging existing health security assets across geographies of import are critical to securing both the health and geopolitical security of member nations. Greater engagement across 'Five Eyes' with a view to cementing health security as a vehicle of strategic and operational influence in key geographies is a pragmatic approach given the escalation of hostilities in a range of critical global settings in which 'Five Eyes' is already operating.

Information Warfare and Cyber-Biological Threats

The manipulation of the online terrain by hostile state and non-state actors reached a new height during the pandemic. Further hostile activity online has centred on cyber-threat activity targeting infrastructure such as the health sector and vaccine research alongside the manipulation of information via pandemic-related disinformation.

Health disinformation, particularly the campaigns waged in recent years by the Kremlin have already compromised essential health and scientific programmes (Bernard et al. 2021b). At the onset of the Russian invasion, Ukraine was the least vaccinated country in Europe against COVID-19 after years of targeted information warfare levelled against immunisation programmes for measles and other vaccine preventable diseases (Bowsher 2022). Russia's triggering of Article V of the Biological Weapons Convention following its spurious disinformation campaigns regarding US biolabs reflects its commitment to undermine international solidarity on vital disarmament regimes using health security and biological research as a narrative lever (Lentzos & Littlewood 2022). Chinese activities have centred on narratives pushing blame for the emergence of COVID-19 outside of China and undermining support for Western vaccines (Hemmings & Varnish 2021). Further disinformation campaigns by non-state actors such as Boko Haram, Al Qaeda, Far Right Groups such as the Proud Boys, and criminal gangs such as MS13 characterise an increasingly diverse and hostile health disinformation ecosystem (Babb & Wilner 2021; Atrache et al. 2020).

In addition to the health of populations, the health sectors of 'Five Eyes' nations have been targeted during the pandemic. Agencies including the NSA, CSIS and GCHQ have publicly acknowledged their efforts countering cyber threat activity directed at State-led cyber-attacks on COVID-19 vaccination programmes (Bell 2020; Fisher and Smyth 2020). During pandemic disruption, criminal actors latched onto the value of health data as a profitable focus of online activity. Cyber-attacks on health sectors such as the Waikato District Health Board in New Zealand have compromised services such as oncology, COVID-19 vaccination and emergency care resulting in patient harm and significant service disruption (Joyce et al. 2021). Following the 2017 Wannacry attack on the UK's National Health Service, calls were made to advance cyber protections for critical health infrastructure, however the escalation of cyber-biological risks outpaced the efforts of 'Five Eyes' members (HoC 2018, Bernard et al. 2021b). At the onset of the pandemic, the realisation that health sector vulnerabilities were placing populations at risk catalysed a rapid re-direction of effort from national intelligence communities towards this relatively neglected sector.

COVID-19 drove an explosion of cyber-biological threats that has generated an unprecedented public response from 'Five Eyes' (Bernard et al. 2020). In a 2020 joint Ministerial Statement, 'Five Eyes' Ministers reflected on the way that 'criminals and hostile actors are exploiting this increased online activity capitalizing on anxieties about the pandemic' and reaffirmed their commitment to cooperation (Australian Government 2020). The tasking of intelligence agencies in all Five nations on these threats has marked a crucial joint venture (Bell 2020). Anticipating that future biological emergencies will be associated with cyber-biological campaigns led by hostile state and non-state actors is a key area upon which 'Five Eyes' can consolidate activity. Building on existing joint 'Five Eyes' consensus to deliver concrete operational interventions will be necessary to accomplish sustained progress against this complexifying threat landscape.

Climate Security and One Health

One of the critical drivers of zoonotic risks (pathogens transmitted between animal and human populations) is the growing impact of climate change, which can drive spillover events by altering equilibria across ecosystem, animal and human domains. Deemed a security priority by the UK Government and described in the 2022 US National Security Strategy as 'the existential challenge of our time', climate change and health security risks increasingly intersect as risk multipliers as they shift from the periphery to the centre of security agendas.

One Health is becoming a dominant paradigm to understand relationships between ecological, social and biological drivers of disease. The 2021 G7 meeting of world leaders pressed the need to develop approaches to improve and strengthen capabilities for One Health horizon scanning and intelligence (G7 2021). Zoonotic diseases such as SARS-CoV-2, Ebola and the MERS have demonstrated the volatility of this space as well as the lack of durable international infrastructure for combatting pandemic threats. The majority of epi- and pandemics originate in animals before spilling over into humans, however the lack of integrated surveillance and poor international animal health governance means emerging infections are poorly monitored across animal species globally. A joint statement by President Biden and former British Prime Minister, Boris Johnson committed to strengthen surveillance and genomic sequencing capabilities to tackle *'variants of concern and emerging infectious disease threats with pandemic or epidemic potential..(by) adopt(ing) a One Health approach to account for animal health, and zoonotic and environmental risk'*. Multilateral international engagement in this space has been coalescing around the biothreat dimensions of One Health risks, driven in part by Canada's Weapons Threat Reduction Programme (WTRP) and the G7-led Global

Partnership against the Spread of Weapons and Materials of Mass Destruction (GP), which have been operating at the One Health-health security interface to support capacity-building activities strengthening public health functions and promoting health security intelligence capabilities.

The US Government has also acknowledged that the Russian invasion of Ukraine hastens the need to move away from fossil fuels – a shift which may produce dividends in both climate and health security terms. As 'Five Eyes' Governments coordinate their efforts on energy security, independent efforts to address climate and health security risks gather pace across the alliance. The UK Health Security Agency (UKHSA) launched a centre for Climate and Health in October 2022, and the US CDC maintains a programme on this theme operating across cities, states, tribes and territories. Opportunity for further 'Five eyes' cooperation on this atypical dimension of contemporary security agendas requires imaginative thinking; in the same way that some scholars have called for 'Five Eyes' interagency working groups or collaborating centres on emerging technologies, so too does this crosscutting issue warrant a joined-up approach, which capitalises on the immense scientific and multilateral capabilities already in place.

Conclusion

Intelligence and health security communities overlap far more than has been publicly acknowledged. COVID-19 has been transformative for driving intelligence sectors to affirm varied taskings and innovations in intersectoral practice. Addressing health security within these intelligence matrices can no longer be seen as a peripheral concern, rather a cross-cutting security issue of significance across 'Five Eyes' (Bowsher and Sullivan 2021a). As the nature of health security threats increasingly centres on the cross-border dimensions of accidental, deliberate or natural infectious diseases, so too have intelligence methods and infrastructure flourished across multilateral networks and in both traditional and non-traditional sectors.

Looking ahead, 'Five Eyes' faces immense challenges, of which the health security intelligence priority is only one. Nevertheless, the pandemic has raised vital questions over the meaning and purpose of collective security, which have only been cemented by overlapping and intersecting crises. International security orders such as NATO and 'Five Eyes' are rightly considering their commitments in financial, existential and ethical terms. The lessons of COVID-19, however, caution against short memories and short-termism, which contributed to the relatively poor performance of some 'Five Eyes' Nations in their own COVID-19 responses. The crisis has provided an opportunity to build upon collective approaches to increasingly complex threat landscapes to support even greater sharing of intelligence on consensus themes. Collaboration on health security intelligence through developing coherent 'counter' approaches' will extend the role of 'Five Eyes' in the health security ecosystem by strengthening core infrastructure, but it will also bolster key existing programmes of work from information and influence operations, to cyber defences, and geostrategic realignment. Ongoing forensic attention towards gaps, failures and opportunities is vital to strengthen future health security intelligence operations in 'Five Eyes' and beyond.

Note

1 The 'biosphere' refers to the region of the earth's surface, sea and air that is inhabited by living organisms.

References

Albert CD, Baez AA, Hunter L, Heslen J, Rutland J (2023) Epidemiological intelligence fusion centers: Health security and COVID-19 in the Dominican Republic. *Intelligence Nat Security*. 38(1), 90–110.

Allam Z (2020) The Rise of Machine Intelligence in the Covid-19 Pandemic and Its Impact on Health Policy. Surveying the COVID-19 Pandemic and Its Implications: 89–96. doi: 10.1016/B978-0-12-824313-8.00006-1. Epub 2020 Jul 24. PMCID: PMC7378493

ASEAN (2021) ASEAN Health Sector Efforts in the Prevention, Detection and Response to Coronavirus Disease 2019 (COVID-19). https://asean.org/asean-health-sector-efforts-in-the-preventiondetection-and-response-to-coronavirus-disease-2019-covid-19-1/

Atrache A, Bentley A, Lamarch A, Schmidtke R (2020) The Coronavirus has become the terrorists' combat weapon of choice. *Refugees International*, June 15. www.refugeesinternational.org/the-coronavirus-has-become-terrorists-combat-weapon-of-choice/

Australian Government (2019) Health Security Initiative for the Indo-Pacific region. https://indopacifichealthsecurity.dfat.gov.au/strategic-framework-2019-2022

Australian Government (2020) Joint Statement Five Eyes Defence Ministers Meeting 23rd June. www.minister.defence.gov.au/statements/2020-06-23/joint-statement-five-eyes-defence-ministers-meeting

Babb W (2021) *Stress Tested: The COVID-19 Pandemic and Canadian National Security*. University of Calgary Press, 33.

Baker M, Baker J, Canyon D, Kevin S (2021) A Biodefense Fusion Center to improve disease surveillance early warnings to improve national security. Daniel K. Inouye Asia Pacific Center for Security Studies, Security Nexus Perspectives. https://dkiapcss.edu/wp-content/uploads/2021/09/2545-Canyon-Network-of-Maritime-Fusion-Centers-v4.pdf

Bell S (2020, December 3) CSIS Accuses Russian, China and Iran of Spreading COVID-19 Disinformation. https://globalnews.ca/news/7494689/csis-accuses-russia-china-iran-coronavirus-covid-19-disinformation/

Bernard R, Bowsher G, Milner C, Boyle P, Patel P, Sullivan R (2018) Intelligence and global health: Assessing the role of open source and social media intelligence analysis in infectious disease outbreaks. *Z Gesundh Wiss*. 26(5): 509–514.

Bernard R, Bowsher G, Sullivan R, Gibson-Fall (2021a) Disinformation and epidemics: Anticipating the next phase of Biowarfare. *Health Secur*. 19(1): 3–12.

Bernard R, Bowsher G, Sullivan R (2021b) Cyber Security and the unexplored threat to global health: A call for global norms. *Global Secur Health Sci Policy*. 5(1): 134–141.

Bernard R, Sullivan R (2020) The use of HUMINT in epidemics: A practical assessment. *Intelligence Natl Secur*. 35(4): 493–501.

Bernardik R, Bowsher G, Sullivan R (2020) COVID-19 and the rise of participatory SIGINT: An examination of the rise in government surveillance through mobile applications. *Am J Public Health*. 110(12): 1780–1785.

Bowsher G (2021) Strengthening cooperation on health security intelligence across the five eyes alliance. Vimy Paper. Conference of Defence Associations Institute. November 2021.

Bowsher G, Bernard R, Sullivan R (2020) A health intelligence framework for pandemic response: Lessons from the UK experience of COVID-19. *Health Secur.* 18(6):435–443.

Bowsher G, Sullivan R (2021) Why we need an intelligence-led approach to pandemics: Supporting science and public health during COVID-19 and beyond. *J R Soc Med.* 114(1):12–14.

Brewster M. (2021) Military medical intelligence warnings gathered dust as public health struggled to define COVID-19. *CBC*, January 11. www.cbc.ca/news/politics/covid-milit ary-medical-intelligence-1.5866627

Bricknell M, Horne S (2020) Personal view: Security sector health systems and global health. *BMJ Mil Health.* Published Online First: 30 September.

Briggs CM, Matejova M, Weiss R (2022) Disaster intelligence: Developing strategic warning for national security. *Intelligence Natl Secur.* 37: 7, 985–1002. https://dx.doi. org/10.1080/02684527.2022.2043080

Bronskill, J (2020) COVID-19 a 'failure of early warning' for Canada, intelligence expert says. *CTV News*, April 13. www.ctvnews.ca/politics/covid-19-a-failure-of-earlywarning-for-canada-intelligence-expert-says-1.4893558

Cabinet Office (2021) Global Britain in a Competitive Age: Integrated Review of Security, Defence, Development and Foreign Policy. https://assets.publishing.service.gov.uk/gov ernment/uploads/system/uploads/attachment_data/file/975077/Global_Britain_in_a_ Competitive_Age_the_Integrated_Review_of_Security__Defence__Development_and_ Foreign_Policy.pdf –

Chertoff M, Bury P, Hatlebrekke K (2020) National intelligence and the Coronavirus Pandemic. *RUSI*, March 31. https://rusi.org/explore-our-research/publications/comment ary/national-intelligence-and-coronavirus-pandemic

Collins HM, Evans R (2002) The third wave of science studies: Studies of expertise and experience. *Soc Stud Sci.* 32(2): 235–296.

CSE (Communications Security Establishment) (2020) *Joint CSE and CSIS Statement – May 14 2020*. Government of Canada. www.canada.ca/en/security-intelligenceservice/ news/2020/05/joint-cse-and-csis-statement.html (last accessed 12/7/2022)

Daoudi S (2020) *The War on COVID-19: The 9/11 of Health Security*. Policy Center for the New South. www.africaportal.org/publications/war-covid-19-911-health-security/

Dahl EJ (2023) *The COVID-19 Intelligence Failure: Why Warning Was Not Enough.* Georgetown University Press.

Davis J (2020) Intelligence, surveillance and ethics in a Pandemic. *Just Security*, 31 March 2020. –www.justsecurity.org/69384/intelligence-surveillance-and-ethics-in-apandemic/

Davis J (2021) Surveillance, intelligence and ethics in a COVID-19 world. In *National Security Intelligence and Ethics*, ed. by Miller S, Regan, M and Walsh PF (pp. 156–166). Routledge.

Department of Justice (2020) Virtual Five Country Ministerial Meeting – Joint Communique, June 26, 2020.

DNI (2021) Annual Meeting of the Five Eyes Intelligence Oversight and Review Council Hosted by the Office of the Inspector-General of Intelligence and Security. New Zealand, November 8–10.

Evans R (2022) SAGE advice and political decision-making: 'Following the science' in times of epistemic uncertainty. *Soc Stud Sci.* 52(1): 53–78.

Fisher L, Smyth C (2020) GCHQ in cyber-war on vaccine Propaganda. *The Times*. www. thetimes.co.uk/article/gchq-in-cyberwar-on-anti-vaccine-propaganda-mcjgjhmb2

Freedman L (2020) Scientific advice at a time of emergency. SAGE and COVID-19. *Polit Q.* 91(3): 514–522.

G7 (2021) Health Ministers' Communique. Carbis Bay Summit, November 2021.

G7 Leaders' Statement on COVID-19 (2020) UK Government, 16 March. www.gov.uk/gov ernment/news/g7-leaders-statement-on-covid-19

Heilweil R (2020) How AI is battling the coronavirus outbreak. *Vox*, January 28. www.vox. com/recode/2020/1/28/21110902/artificial-intelligence-ai-coronavirus-wuhan

Hemmings J, Varnish P (2021) Evolving the 5 Eyes. Opportunities and Challenges in. the New Strategic Landscape. https://macdonaldlaurier.ca/files/pdf/20210913_Five_ Eyes_Hemmings_Varnish_PAPER_FWeb.pdf

HM Government (2018) *UK Biological Security Strategy*. The Home Office. https://assets. publishing.service.gov.uk/government/uploads/system/uploads/attachment_data/file/730 213/2018_UK_ Biological_Security_Strategy.pdf (last accessed 15/9/2020)

HM Government (2023) *UK Biological Security Strategy*. Cabinet Office. https://assets. publishing.service.gov.uk/media/64c0ded51e10bf000e17ceba/UK_Biological_Security_ Strategy.pdf

House of Commons Select Committee (2018) *Faster Action Needed on Lessons of Wannacry Attack.* www.parliament.uk/ business/committees/committees-a-z/commons- select/ public-accounts-committee/news-parliament-2017/nhs-cyber-attack-report- published-17-19/

IPPPR (2021) COVID-19: Make it the Last Pandemic by The Independent Panel for Pandemic Preparedness & Response https://theindependentpanel.org/wpcontent/

Janeva A, Harris A, Byrne J (2022) The future of open source intelligence for UK national security. *RUSI Occasional Paper.* https://static.rusi.org/330_OP_FutureOfOpenSourc eIntelligence_FinalWeb0.pdf

Jarman H, Rozenblum S, Falkenbach M, Rockwell O, Greer SL (2022) Role of scientific advice in covid-19 policy. *BMJ.* 378: 1–4.

Joyce C, Roman L, Miller B, Jeffries J, Miller RC (2021) Emerging cybersecurity threats in radiation oncology. *Adv Rad Oncol.* 6(6): 100796.

Lakoff A (2018) *Unprepared: Global Health in a Time of Emergency*. University of California Press.

Lentzos F, Goodman G (2020) Health security intelligence: Engaging across disciplines and sectors. *Intelligence Natl Secur.* 35(4): 465–476.

Lentzos, F, Littlewood, J (2022, July 8) Russian finds another stage for the Ukraine 'Biolabs' disinformation show. *Bulletin of the Atomic Scientists*, 1–11. https://thebulletin.org/2022/ 07/russia-finds-another-stage-for-the-ukraine-biolabs-disinformation-show/#post-head ing (last accessed 28/8/2022)

Levy A, Wark W (2021, July 23) *The Pandemic Caught Canada Unawares: It Was an Intelligence Failure.* Centre for International Governance Innovation. www.cigionline. org/ articles/the-pandemic-caught-canada-unawares-it-was-an-intelligence-failure/

Manancourt V, Scott M (2021) In Europe, a coronavirus boom for foreign surveillance firms. *Politico*, May 28. www.politico.eu/article/europe-surveillance-china-israel-uni ted-states/

Markson S (2021) *What Really Happened in Wuhan*. Harper Collins.

Migliore L, Hopkins D, Jumpp S, Brackett C, Cromheecke J (2021) Medical intelligence team lessons learned: Early activation and knowledge product development mitigate COVID-19 Threats. *Military Med.* 186(2): 15–22.

National Intelligence Council (2022) National Intelligence Estimate NIE 2022–02480, Economics and National Security Implications of the COVID-19 Pandemic through 2026.

National Intelligence Estimate NIE 2022–02480 (Declassified January 2023). www.dni. gov/files/ODNI/documents/assessments/NIE-Economic_and_National_Securtiy_Implic ations_of_the_COVID-19_Pandemic_Through_2026.pdf

Niiler E (2020) An AI epidemiologist sent the first warnings of the Wuhan Virus. *Wired.* www.wired.com/story/ai-epidemiologist-wuhan-public-health-warnings/

Omand D (2020) Will the intelligence agencies spot the next outbreak. *The Article*, May 18. www.thearticle.com/will-the-intelligence-agencies-spot-the-next-outbreak

Pfeifer J (2012) Network fusion: Information and intelligence sharing for a networked world. *Homeland Security Affairs.* 8(17): 1–20.

Pfluke C (2019) A history of the five eyes alliance: Possibility for reform and additions. *Comp Strategy.* 38(4): 302–315.

PHAC (2023) *Health Portfolio Emergency Response Plan.* Government of Canada. www. canada.ca/en/public-health/services/publications/health-risks-safety/health-portfolio-emergency-response-plan.html#a2

PHAC Independent Review Panel (2021) *Global Public Health Intelligence Network (GPHIN) Review Panel Final Report.* www.canada.ca/en/public-health/corporate/mand ate/aboutagency/

Reuters (2022) Brazilian firm to make Russia's Sputnik Light COVID vaccine for export. *Reuters*, February 17. www.reuters.com/business/healthcare-pharmaceuticals/brazilian-firm-make-russias-sputnik-light-covid-vaccine-export-2022-02-17/

Sengupta K (2020) Coronavirus: British Army Called into Help Quash Online Conspiracy Theories. May 30 . www.independent.co.uk/independentpremium/uk-news/british-army coronavirus-conspiracy-theory-5g-a9538791.html

Shapira (2020) Israeli National Intelligence and the Response to COVID-19. War on The Rocks. November 20 . https://warontherocks.com/2020/11/israeli-national-intelligence culture-and-the-response-to-covid-19/

The White House (2022 September) US COVID-19 Global Response & Recovery Framework. www.whitehouse.gov/wp-content/uploads/2022/09/U.S.-COVID-19-GLO BAL-RESPONSE-RECOVERY-FRAMEWORK-_clean_9-14_7pm.pdf

UKHSA (2024) www.gov.uk/government/organisations/uk-health-security-agency#:~:text= The%20UK%20Health%20Security%20Agency%20(UKHSA)%20is%20responsi ble%20for%20protecting,incidents%20and%20other%20health%20threats.

Vickery J, Atkinson P, Lin L, Rubin O, Upshur R, Yeoh EK, Boyer C, Errett NA (2022) Challenges to evidence-informed decision-making in the context of pandemics: Qualitative study of COVID-19 policy advisor perspectives. *BMJ Glob Health.* 7(4): e008268.

Walsh P (2014) Building better intelligence frameworks through effective governance. *Int J Intelligence Counterintelligence.* 28(1): 123–142.

Walsh P (2020a) *Building a Better Pandemic and Health Security Intelligence Response in Australia.* CIGI.

Walsh P (2020b) Improving 'five eyes' health security intelligence capabilities: Leadership and governance challenges. *Intelligence Natl Secur.* 35(4): 586–602.

Walsh PF (2023) Australia's national intelligence community: Challenges and opportunities in a multi-polar world. In *Intelligence Cooperation under Multipolarity: Non American Perspectives*, ed. by Juneau T, Massie J and Munier M. University of Toronto Press.

Walton C (2020). Spies Are Fighting a Shadow War Against the Coronavirus Foreign Policy. April 3, 2020.

Wark W (2020, March) *Health Intelligence, National Security and the COVID-19 Pandemic.* Canadian Global Affairs Institute. https://d3n8a8pro7vhmx.cloudfront.net/cdfai/pages/4399/attachments/original/1585597305/Health_Intelligence__National_Security_and_the_COVID-19_Pandemic.pdf?1585597305

West L, Juneau T, Amarasingham A (2021) *Stress Tested: The COVID-19 Pandemic and Canadian National Security.* University of Calgary Press.

Wilson JM, Lake CK, Matthews M, Southard M, Leone R, McCarthy M (2022) Health security warning intelligence during first contact with COVID: An operations perspective. *Intelligence Natl Secur.* 37(2): 216–240.

Wilson JW, McNamara T (2020) The 1999 West Nile virus warning signal revisited. *Intelligence Natl Secur.* 35(4): 519–526.

Young G (2020) Defence chief says 77 Brigade is countering COVID misinformation. *The National,* April 22.

Zarocostas J (2020) How to fight an infodemic. *Lancet.* 395(10225): 676.

Zegart A (2023) Ukraine and the next intelligence revolution. *Foreign Affairs,* January/February (pre-press). www.foreignaffairs.com/world/open-secrets-ukraine-intelligence-revolution-amyzegart?utm_campaign=ln_daily_soc&utm_source=linkedIn_posts&utm_medium=social

Zenko, M (2020) The Coronavirus is the worst intelligence failure in US history. *Foreign Policy.* 25(3). https://foreignpolicy.com/2020/03/25/coronavirus-worst-intelligence-failureus-history-covid-19/

6 Improving Health Security Intelligence Warning Systems

David Skillicorn

Introduction

The technical challenges of developing an automated health intelligence warning system can be summarised in these three key questions:

- Which indicators should be attended to?
- When does an indicator's value become significant (that is, when does an indicator produce an indication)?
- How should significant indications be combined to become actionable?

In a health context, indicators can be of many kinds: pathogen related (genetic changes), public health related (case counts), social (behaviours associated with transmission), social media (misinformation, denial), infrastructure (PPE supply, sampling capacity, vaccination capacity), political (funding levels), international (misinformation, espionage), and climate (heatwaves).

The requirements of intelligence warning systems make answering these key questions difficult. The initial indications of never-before-seen events often do not seem important. For example, in the COVID-19 pandemic, the importance of social media in spreading misinformation or of criminal activity in misappropriating government funding and stealing PPE was not anticipated. Most indicators in intelligence settings are *weak or uncertain* – any individual indicator's values at a particular moment can seem like noise, an outlier, a glitch along the collection pathway, or in some other way insignificant (Ansoff 1975; Holopainen and Toivonen 2012). Situational awareness, sensemaking, and deciding to act require noticing and combining the values of multiple weak indications, appropriately weighted, to create a strong indication.

Approaches to detecting and integrating weak or uncertain indicators have been developed in business (Ojala and Uskall 2006; Schoemaker and Day 2009; Kima and Lee 2017), health (Veerman et al. 2007; Macrae 2014), information security (Kajava et al. 2005), counterterrorism (Papachristos 2009; Bryniellsson et al. 2013; Beardsley and Beech 2013; Koivisto et al. 2016; Andrews et al. 2018; Dudenhofer et al. 2021), and policing (Vogt 2017). These papers are, however, almost all abstract (surveys of the space of solutions) or anecdotal. Computational work exists, for

DOI: 10.4324/9781003335511-9

example Andrews et al. (2001) and Brynielsson et al. (2013) but these systems consider only indicators arising from natural language content, for example posts by potential lone-wolf terrorists, and use relatively simple bag-of-words approaches. The state-of-the-art even in well-developed intelligence warning systems is still patchy.

Some health systems, for example Epiwatch (www.epiwatch.org/map) process many millions of online documents, and extract mentions of diseases or syndromes, making them available as geographical counts. However, most of the situational awareness is left to analysts who must notice changes in the pattern of counts. One of the subtle drawbacks of such systems is that online documents are mostly written about surprising occurrences. This is exactly what is needed for health intelligence early warning, but the difficulty is that there is typically no baseline for a disease or syndrome because 'ordinary' occurrences do not get written about. So, for example, there may be documents written at the beginning of 'flu season' but, unless the case rates are unusual, there tend to be few documents written during it.

Figure 6.1 shows an example of the output of Epiwatch, in this case for Australia in (Southern) Winter of 2023 for three selected diseases. Despite being the middle of 'flu season' the number of dark black shaded each with a value of '1' (ILI) is very small and provides no sense of the progress of the season.

There are also some developments in process control, where the kind of warning systems we are talking about here are sometimes called dynamic risk assessment (Paltrinieri and Khan 2016). Pasman (2020) surveys some examples of the failures of warning systems and makes the point that failures are sometimes the fault of those who should have heeded the warnings rather than the warning system itself.

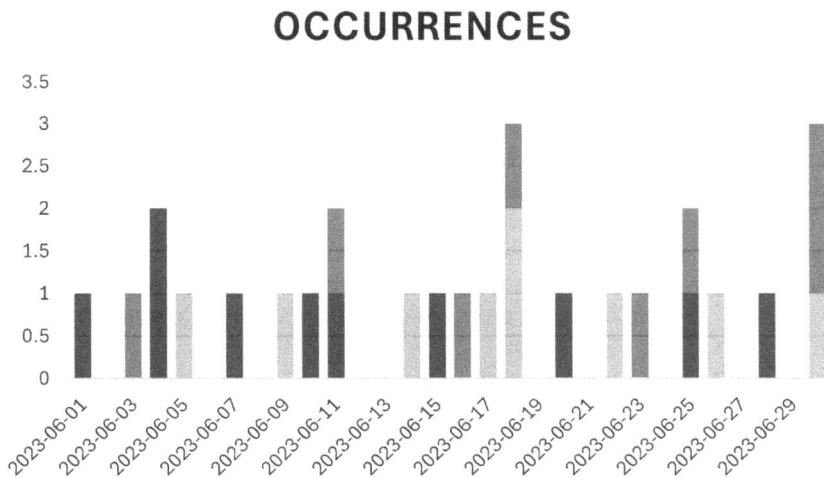

Figure 6.1 Each block is a mention of a particular disease or syndrome on a particular day.

Source: Generated by author using data derived from Epiwatch.

The risk literature, of course, has tried to detect risks and adverse events, but they have typically focused on risks that are straightforward to quantify, for example by actuarial models. There is growing acknowledgement of more serious categories of anomalous events that would previously have been regarded as too unlikely for consideration and action: gray rhinos (Wucker 2016), catastrophes whose likelihood is high and visible, but for which preventive actions are still not taken; black swans (Taleb 2010), unpredictable, rare catastrophic events; and dragon kings (Sornette and Ouillon 2012), unique, high-impact catastrophes. The discussions of these classes of events are still rather abstract and computational approaches to detecting any of them are limited. However, in the wake of the COVID-19 pandemic and several substantial financial crises, the banking sector has become much readier to face the possibility of catastrophic events and to incorporate these into their risk modelling.

Intelligence systems also face a particular problem: there are adversaries who are deliberately trying to break the ability to respond in a timely and appropriate way by corrupting the data collected, and by creating artificial indicator values (both too low to suppress attention, and too high to create false alarms until users learn to ignore the system outputs). This is less of a problem for health intelligence systems that collect data about disease activity itself. However, there is often considerable overlap between systems to warn of health issues and mainstream intelligence warning systems – for example, the use of anthrax in the aftermath of the 9/11 attacks, the manipulation of social media during the COVID-19 pandemic to create fear and have political effects, and the cyberespionage aimed at stealing intellectual property related to vaccines. Even health intelligence warning systems must be aware of a possible adversarial dimension.

The ideal intelligence warning system would be a kind of dashboard that shows both the values of each indicator and an integration into an overall situational awareness model. In security intelligence settings, this is still largely a human-driven process in which information is collected by analysts who try to make sense of it, decide which parts are most salient, and integrate them into an intelligence brief that represents the current moment. Systems such as Palantir (www.palantir.com/) provide some tool support for this task, enabling data to be presented and manipulated in subtle ways to assist analysts to make sense of it, and to ensure that important parts are not ignored. However, such systems are assistants for human analysts rather than tools that directly warn of developing dangerous situations. The skill of analysts deciding what information to collect, how to assess and weight it, and how to integrate disparate pieces into an actionable whole remains key to the process.

Health intelligence warning systems are not, at present, so sophisticated. Most countries have some form of disease early-warning system, but the COVID-19 pandemic showed that these are often too sluggish to respond to exponentially increasing cases, and struggle with multiple, incoherent sources of data. There are some exceptions: the Acute Care Enhanced Surveillance system (www.kflaphi.ca/acute-care-enhanced-surveillance/) in Ontario, Canada, collects textual data entered by the triage nurse as each patient arrives at the emergency department at every hospital in the province. It then automatically applies natural-language data-analytic clustering techniques to map the patient into one of 80 syndromes in real time. The current state and rate of change of the syndromes can be viewed from moment to moment by any public health unit in the province. The system was sensitive enough to detect an outbreak of food poisoning early enough to trace it to its source. However, the limitations of such systems are illustrated by the COVID-19 pandemic. Early cases presented with symptoms that overlap with many other diseases (pneumonia, influenza-like illness), and so the ACES system did not immediately detect the local start of the pandemic. Also, the ACES system lives within a single-payer provincial health insurance system and so the data collection is consistent and mandatory. In more complex environments such as the U.S., a system of this kind would be extremely difficult to deploy because of the patchwork of organisations that would be involved: hospitals, clinics, public health organisations and health insurers, themselves within city, county, state and federal jurisdictions. At international scale the problem is, of course, much more difficult. The World Health Organisation's Epidemic Intelligence from Open Sources system detected the first document about an unusual cluster of pneumonia in Wuhan on 31 December 2019, but many weeks passed before this early indicator led to action. The first case outside China was detected on 13 January 2020, but it was not until 14 January that the World Health Organization indicated that there might have been human-to-human transmission. A pandemic was not declared until 11 March, by which time many countries were on the brink of lockdowns. Retrospective studies (Macintyre et al. 2023) have shown that COVID-19 could have been detected many days earlier if the right indicators had been available and were being tracked.

Automated or partially automated health intelligence warning systems can assist public health professionals by drawing attention to a changing environment and help to decrease the inertia that often prevents sharp changes from being fully appreciated. Health intelligence systems need to warn proactively, especially in a globally connected world, but it seems clear that the World Health Organisation's ethos was to be conservative. Automated systems can help to convince governments of the need for action because the systems themselves cannot be accused of being self serving, and so an aspect of the political dimension is removed from the process. Of course, the best health intelligence warning system is useless if those who could act fail to do so; and such a system must build a robust track record that makes it easier for decision makers to act.

Which Indicators Should Be Attended to?

There is an inherent tension between the cost of collecting as many potential indicators as possible (with the downstream computational cost of processing them) and the blind spots from missing indicators that turn out to be important. Recent health cases have made the point. The COVID-19 pandemic showed that, with the best will in the world, many important indicators were not, and often could not, be collected. Case counts, hospitalisations and deaths could not be accurately measured (and still cannot after several years), even in Western countries with strong health systems (Alvarez et al. 2023). The Mpox epidemic could perhaps have been reduced if a significant indicator had not been missed: the sudden increase in rate of mutations of the virus in West Africa. This fact had been observed, but its potential importance was not (Scientific American 2022). It is inherently difficult to tell, in advance, which indicators will turn out to be critical in predicting a significantly changing risk or an adverse event (Ansoff 1975). The conservative strategy, therefore, is to err on the side of collecting more indicators but, in a public health environment, cost is typically a more important issue than coverage.

When Does an Indicator's Value Become Significant?

Before the significance of an indicator can be assessed, its properties must be understood, including:

- Its provenance. The source of each indicator and its reliability need to be understood before any other judgement can be made about it. Indicators may come from: physical devices such as temperature sensors or other Internet-of-Things devices, digital data such as counts of emergency visits to a hospital, outputs of data-analytic models such as natural-language analysis of online posts, or anecdotal information from discussions among physicians. All have potential sources of unreliability. A temperature sensor may have a hardware failure or may be in direct sun during part of the day; some hospitals may not provide counts of emergency visits on weekends or may silently aggregate multiple days. Attempts to assess influenza-like illness (ILI) using online mentions (a system once used by Google) can founder because of the use of 'flu' to describe many different, even non-respiratory, illnesses; and anecdotes are, by their nature, sparse data. This is further complicated by the possibility of adversaries deliberately trying to corrupt the data being collected.
- The relationship of indicator magnitude to semantics. We have become accustomed to the magnitudes of common measurements so that it is easy to forget that these magnitudes do not necessarily correspond in a straightforward way to their meanings. Americans travelling internationally can be surprised at the apparently high speed limits, but the surprising cold temperature forecasts – they assume the wrong semantics because of misunderstood magnitudes. Another common measure whose semantics nobody understands well is the probability of precipitation in weather forecasts. What does it mean when there is a 40% chance of rain?

    In every location in the area 40% of the time? In 40% of the locations?

    The decoupling of magnitude from meaning is particularly evident when the indicator is itself the product of some upstream process. For example, it is common for data-analytic predictors to output a value between 0 and 1. However, the magnitude of this predicted value often has little to do with the strength of the prediction, except to the obvious extent that a larger value indicates a prediction of one outcome more than the other. In particular, there is no justification for treating such an output as a probability, although this is often done.

- Its context. The larger system from which the indicator comes must be considered when making judgements about it. Of course, some indicators are designedly independent of their context – a fire alarm is a straightforward indicator that everyone is expected to act on. But most other systems have some room for interpretation in the gap between the indicator and a following action. For example, a common mantra in security is 'if you see something, say something'. But individuals hardly ever do say something, and when they do, those they say it to hardly ever act on it. (One of the differences between security organisations and fire fighters is that fire fighters roll on every alarm, while intelligence organisations are much more restrained.) A recent terrorist attack changes the threshold, making it far more likely that individuals will say something and security organisations will take it seriously and a recent pandemic has a similar effect, but these changes are not long lasting (Phillips and Pohl 2020).

  Of course, this dynamic makes it possible for bad actors to conceal their actions using 'the boy who cried wolf' strategy: generating so many false alarms that those who should react stop doing so until eventually a real alarm is ignored. This dynamic can happen even when humans are not involved: a device that continually produces false alarms will eventually be ignored. This strategy has been exploited against high-end burglar alarms; after several false alarms the temptation is strong to turn off the apparently malfunctioning part of the system.

  A single case of Ebola in a country where it is more or less endemic produces a public health response, but not on the scale that a handful of cases of Ebola did when they were detected in the U.S. in 2014 (https://archive.cdc.gov/#/deta ils?url=https://www.cdc.gov/about/ebola/ebola-by-the-numbers.html). It is not usually possible to decide on the meaning of a single indicator's value without some context.

- Rates of change. Many indicators change their values with time, and it may be a second-order effect, the rate of change, that is important. Some change their value in a cyclic way, for example ambient outdoor temperature. This underlying, expected variation must be discounted before it is clear whether a particular change warrants attention. For example, influenza-like illness ('flu') has a characteristic high incidence during the winters in non-equatorial countries. While higher than normal incidence peaks are of interest, peaks outside the normal timeframe are a much more significant indicator.

To determine if an indicator is anomalous, all of these properties must be taken into account: is the indicator reliable, is its value meaningfully unusual, is it unusual in its context, and is it unusual in its time frame? There is a further complication: if an indicator value is slightly unusual then this is probably significant but if it is extremely unusual, it probably is not. For example, if an indoor temperature sensor reads 50°C then this may be significant, but if it reads 5000°C then this is far more likely to be a problem with the sensor. Judging the boundary between unusual and implausible is difficult. One of the takeaways from the COVID-19 pandemic is that most people do not understand exponential growth; they understand that growth can be fast, but not that the rate of growth itself can constantly increase. With 1,000 cases today, a prediction of 4,000 two days away and 16,000 four days away was interpreted as totally implausible, and discounted by many people (Lammers et al. 2020), including public health professionals (www.bbc.com/future/article/20200 812-exponential-growth-bias-the-numerical-error-behind-COVID-19).

In many systems where humans make judgements of anomaly, they rely on experience, perhaps encoded in rules of thumb. A large part of the training of intelligence officers is exactly aimed at developing such judgement. However, a number of high-profile examples – the Challenger disaster, the 9/11 attacks, the invasion of Iraq, the COVID-19 pandemic, and the invasion of Ukraine – show how this process can fail even when the process and the participants are both sophisticated. Rules of thumb are also surprisingly persistent, even in the face of strong contrary evidence. In the first few months of the COVID-19 pandemic, public health responses tended to assume that COVID-19 resembled an influenza-like illness, for which some pandemic preparations had been made and training scenarios had been exercised, even though it quickly became clear that COVID-19 was not at all like ILI. Another example of acting on outdated rules is the Axis confidence, in World War II, that an Allied attack on the European mainland must come through Calais, even after it was clear that a massive landing had already happened in Normandy.

Statisticians have long developed methods for judging significance that are not so vulnerable to human nature. These are mostly answers to questions of the form: how likely is it that this outcome is the product of chance rather than representing an underlying reality? Such methods are routinely used to assess whether experiments have in fact demonstrated what they were designed to do. There are two weaknesses to using these methods in intelligence settings. First, the most interesting situations from an intelligence perspective are one-offs and so general models of significance do not straightforwardly apply. Second, statistical significance testing almost always wires in an assumption of Gaussian or normal distributions, which are representative of many natural-world phenomena but not of those that involve human activity. For example, today's temperature can be estimated from the distribution of temperatures on this day in previous years, which will typically have the bell shape of the Gaussian distribution. However, the number of people with asthma arriving at an emergency department today is much harder to estimate; there will perhaps be a Gaussian component, but it also depends, for example, on the day of the week (since emergency department visits peak on Mondays).

In particular, many human-mediated systems can best be modelled using statistical distributions that are heavy-tailed, that is the probability of cases far from the mean or median is much higher than a Gaussian distribution would indicate. For example, financial market operators such as Nassim Taleb (2010) have argued for decades that real-world systems behave in ways very different from Gaussian, but that risk management techniques persist in using Gaussians because it seems intuitive and makes the analysis more tractable. The difference is illustrated by the joke 'Bill Gates walks into a bar, and suddenly the average net worth of everyone present becomes hundreds of millions of dollars'. The fact that insurance payouts are heavy-tailed (there are occasional extremely large payouts – for a single car, $US1.2 million, hurricane Katrina, $US45 billion, and the collapse of the Lloyd's 'names' in ship insurance, multiple 'hundred year' floods in the past century) shows that the risks of many adverse events must be heavy tailed too.

A robust health intelligence system is most useful when it accurately predicts the most extreme events, but this is not necessarily obvious to the users of such systems. Suppose that, before the COVID-19 pandemic, public health officials were asked if they would prefer an intelligence system that would accurately predict each year's ILI severity, or the start of a pandemic. Most would have chosen the first alternative for what would have seemed obvious reasons: ILI is expensive for health systems but remains quite unpredictable, while pandemics are rare. Even without an explicit preference, the amounts spent on pandemic preparation reflected the perceived low priority of this possibility. And yet, in retrospect, the cost of the COVID-19 pandemic is many orders of magnitude higher than that of ILI for the entire time since the 'Spanish Flu' epidemic of a hundred years ago. The heavy tailed parts of distributions are the most important to model, but they are the easiest to neglect when designing models.

How Should Significant Indicator Values Be Combined to Become Actionable?

One way of compensating for the difficulty of determining when any individual indicator is significant is to consider each indicator against the background of the other available indicators. It is unlikely that any significant event can be seen only in the change in one indicator, so considering the entire set of indicator values at once is an overall better strategy. Each indicator's significance is assessed by considering it against the background of the values of all the other indicators. Of course, there is a circularity here, but it is one that can be addressed computationally.

Suppose that we define the space spanned by all the available indicators and call this a *configuration space*. For example, if a building has two temperature sensors then this space is two-dimensional. The instantaneous outputs of the indicators define a point in this space. This space provides a way to consider how the indicators from the sensors relate to one another, and to the sets of previous indicator values. In other words, there is a context for each of the instantaneous indicator value sets: where the corresponding point lies in the configuration space; but also the history of the sets of indicator values, a trajectory through the configuration space.

In a typical building, each temperature sensor probably reads between 18°C and 25°C but these will vary through the day. Although both sensors will tend to move in a roughly synchronous way, this won't be exact because of differences

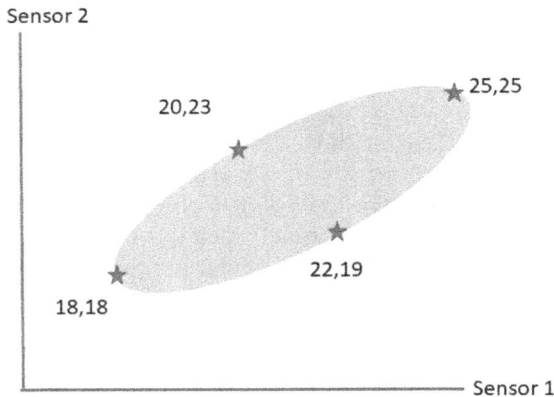

Figure 6.2 Stylised representations of the trajectories of temperatures from two sensors through time.

Source: Author.

in location. Normal patterns will produce a cloud of points in the region bounded by 18 and 25 in each of the two dimensions, but the cloud will be cigar-shaped because a larger value in one sensor tends to be correlated with larger values in the other. Within the cloud there will be a roughly cyclic trajectory reflecting how temperatures increase and decrease through each day. A stylised representation is shown in Figure 6.2. Now if one of the sensors has a much higher reading, say 30°C, then the corresponding point will fall outside the cloud, and the trajectory leading to it will turn, probably sharply. The presence of the cloud makes it easier to see how significant this unusual reading is. The judgement of significance is not made based on a single set of indicator values in isolation, nor even of the historical record of a single indicator, but is instead based on the collective pattern of all of the indicators over all of the historical records. This is a much more robust way to make judgements of significance.

Scaling up this idea faces two challenges. In practice there are many indicators, perhaps hundreds or more, so the dimensionality of the configuration space is high. And the scales of different dimensions are not necessarily comparable, so that the change in an indicator value in one dimension causes a different change in the position of a configuration than a change in an indicator value in another dimension. For example, if we have sensors that measure temperatures in Celsius and relative humidity in percent, then we can define a two-dimensional configuration space for the readings of the two sensors, but the difference between readings of (18°C, 65% humidity) and (20°C, 65% humidity), and between (18°C, 65% humidity) and (18°C, 67% humidity) are not the same, even though each is a change of magnitude 2 in one of the values.

These are not new challenges since they also apply to data-analytic clustering algorithms that also start from the space spanned by the attributes. The key property that we need is to define a meaningful similarity between configurations, because only then can we decide when a particular configuration is dissimilar enough to others to be significant.

The first step is to normalise the indicator values so that all indicators are on the same scale. This is not a completely solvable problem: how should a difference of 2 degrees be compared to a difference of 2 percent relative humidity? The conventional approach is to convert the values of each indicator to z-scores, computing the mean and standard deviation of each dimension and then subtracting the mean and dividing by the standard deviation of each value for that indicator, and using these values instead. This converts the values of each of the indicators into common units of standard deviations which are at least plausibly comparable. This process of using the mean and standard deviation is only an accurate transformation if the values of each indicator are distributed in a Gaussian way and, except for some natural-world properties, this is almost never the case.

This approach also does not work for indicators that have a fixed number of discrete values (say, low, medium, and high), where one common convention is to use one-hot encoding. For example, a hospital admission record might describe, for each patient, a condition or syndrome for which they were admitted. An indicator is associated with each possible syndrome with a 1 for the indicator corresponding to the patient's syndrome and a 0 for all the others. This works reasonably well when the number of possibilities is small but does not scale well. If there are 80 different syndromes, then the original indicator with 80 discrete values ('ILI', 'pneumonia', 'broken bone', ...) has become 80 new indicators. Measuring similarity between patients becomes more difficult because each has only one (or perhaps a few) non-zeroes among these 80 indicators.

For some kinds of qualitative indicators, the same approach (one-hot encoding) can be taken, or the indicator values can be converted to numbers. For example, a terror attack threat level (low, moderate, high, immediate) could be one-hot encoded, or just mapped to the values 1, 2, 3 and 4 because the original levels have an implicit order.

Normalisation is a necessary evil – any plausible computational definition of similarity requires it, but it always introduces artifacts into the configuration space.

Once the configuration space has been normalised, that is its extents along each axis are on the same scale, similarity becomes equivalent to distance: similar configurations are close. It is now straightforward to answer questions like: how unusual is the current configuration (compared to all of the others), and how unusual is it looking back over the trajectory of recent configurations? However, high-dimensional spaces, generated from many indicators, are awkward settings to measure similarity, intuitively because there are so many ways to be dissimilar. It is therefore conventional to reduce the dimensionality by projecting the configuration space into a space of fewer dimensions in a way that preserves as much of its structure as possible. A little surprisingly, reducing the dimensionality often improves the calculation of similarity because it also removes some of the variation among points that is the result of noisy measurements.

If it is sensible to regard the configuration space as linear, that is the dissimilarity between two points (configurations) is represented exactly by the distance between them no matter where they are in the space, then linear dimensionality-reduction techniques are appropriate. These can be thought of as flying a drone around the cloud of points in the high-dimensional representation looking for a viewpoint from which the cloud has the greatest variation. The cloud can then be projected onto the plane of the drone's view, producing a one dimensional smaller representation, and the process repeated. The standard way to do this is to use *singular value decomposition* (Skillicorn 2007), a method that has two advantages. First, it guarantees that a projection into a smaller number of dimensions is the most faithful possible representation of the cloud in that lower dimensionality, that is it guarantees to preserve as much structure as possible. Second, it produces a sorted list in decreasing order of the magnitudes of the variations in each of the new dimensions so that the choice of how many dimensions to use can be informed by knowing exactly how much variation is being discarded by that choice. An example of a dashboard using this idea and applied to intrusion detection in computer systems is found in Skillicorn (2012).

Figure 6.3 shows a configuration space derived from the number of emergency room visits for three syndromes: ILI, an infectious disease, asthma, caused by a combination of genetics and environmental triggers, and COPD, caused by long-term exposure to lung irritants, over the period of a year. The figure shows one point

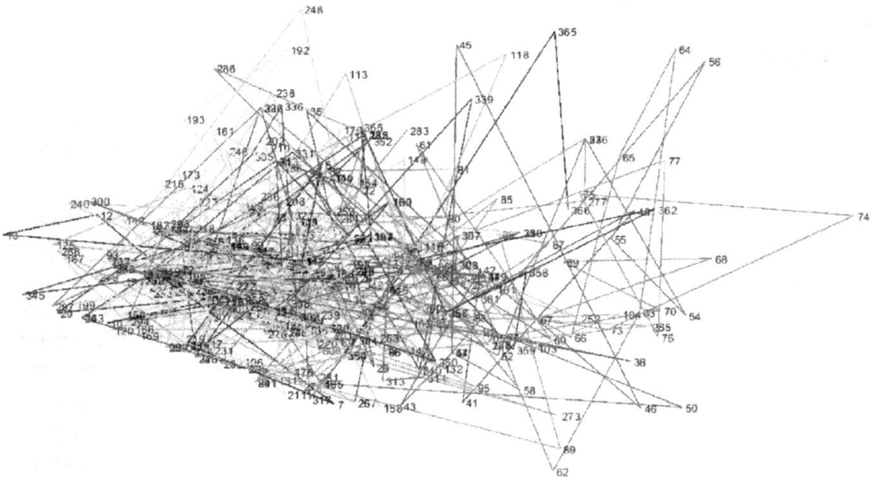

Figure 6.3 Trajectory of daily emergency room visit counts for ILI, asthma and COPD over one year in a linear configuration space.

Source: Author.

for each day, numbered by the day of the year it represents, with lines connecting adjacent days whose colours get darker through the year.

The points on the right-hand end of the configuration space are for dates primarily in February and March. This is entirely expected for ILI which, in the Northern Hemisphere, peaks at this time of year, but it is surprising to see that incidence of asthma and COPD are correlated with ILI but only during this period. In the remainder of the year, the counts of the three syndromes are uncorrelated. This is probably explainable by invoking either increased time spent inside, and so greater exposure to triggers, or increased exposure to other respiratory viruses causing breathing distress as side effects. But the need for an explanation at all would not have been visible without the configuration space representation of the data.

The similarity between two configurations may not be best captured simply by the distance between them. For example, the difference between a newborn baby and a two-year-old is a significant difference, but the difference between a 60-year-old and a 62-year-old is not, despite both being a gap of two years. For temperatures, a gap of 2 degrees is usually not significant, except if the gap is between $+1°$ and $-1°$. The cloud of points (configurations) may form a spiral, so that some points may be quite close to one another in distance but obviously on different parts of the spiral. A reasonable way to compute similarity should take into account properties of the neighbourhood, not just the distance between two points in isolation. In cases like this, a non-linear dimensionality-reduction technique is more useful.

Non-linear dimensionality-reduction uses, broadly speaking, two different techniques. The first turns the set of points into a (mathematical) graph by joining pairs of points by an edge weighted by how similar the two corresponding indicators are, usually with a threshold so that pairs that are only weakly similar do not get connected. This results in an abstract structure, the graph, rather than the configuration space. This abstract structure can be embedded in a new, low-dimensional space that reflects its structure using *spectral embedding* (von Luxburg 2007). The embedding technique is akin to singular value decomposition so that the choice of dimensionality can be made knowing how much structure is being ignored by discarding some dimensions.

The second technique uses neural-network-based clustering algorithms to represent the non-linear similarities. Some of the choices are t-SNE (van der Maaten and Hinton 2008), (variational) autoencoders (Kingman and Welling 2019), radial basis neural networks (Hwang and Bang 1997), or a number of other deep-learning approaches (Arvanitidis et al. 2012). These techniques are relatively new, so there is no consensus about which technique is best. Most of them also have many parameters so it can require considerable experimentation to find good low-dimensional representations.

Although configuration spaces are appealing, and perhaps even necessary as ways to represent anomalies, the state-of-the-art from data analytics is still underdeveloped. Linear configuration spaces are better understood, but their use for anomaly detection is patchy. Nonlinear configuration spaces are even less well understood. These are active research areas in data analytics.

One glaring omission in the research in this area is the application of Bayesian concepts. The central Bayesian idea is that the relevance of some piece of data or evidence to a conclusion must also depend on the base probability of that conclusion, its prior probability or just prior. In a simple example, suppose that flashing lights are observed in the sky at night. What are the chances that they are caused by invading aliens? To estimate the answer correctly it is important to know how likely it is to see flashing lights in the sky at night (quite likely) *and* how likely it is that aliens are invading, in the absence of any information (extremely unlikely). The product of these two likelihoods is small, so we conclude that the flashing lights almost certainly do not mean aliens are invading. The likelihood that planes are flying overhead at night is moderate in the absence of other information, so the product of these two likelihoods – quite likely flashing lights and moderately likely planes – is moderate, so we conclude that that the lights are plausibly associated with planes.

Conspiracy theorists often acquire their ideas because they ignore the important role of priors and concentrate instead on evidence alone, thereby giving it much greater weight than it would otherwise have. But many others who are not conspiracy theorists are also fooled by failing to think about priors. Suppose that a medical test has a diagnostic accuracy of 80% and a patient has a positive test. What is the chance that she actually has the disease? Many practitioners will say that it is 80%; after all the test misses only 20% of the cases. But the correct answer also depends on the base rate for the disease, that is what is the chance that anyone chosen at random has the disease. Suppose for simplicity that the base rate is 10%, so 10 in a hundred have the disease. If one hundred patients are tested, then 8 out of 10 of those who actually have the disease will test positive and 2 will test negative. For the other 90, 72 will test negative, but 20% of them, 18, will test positive. So, of the 26 who tested positive, 8 actually have the disease but 18 do not, so the chance that the patient with a positive test actually has the disease is $8/26 = 0.31 = 31\%$. This is much smaller than 80%! If the base rate were much smaller, then almost all the positive tests would be false positives. In other words, it is really difficult to detect inherently rare events.

For a health intelligence system, a Bayesian approach is a more formal way to consider the role of context. There has been little research on how to include Bayesian ideas into detecting unusual events. Roberts et al. (2022) develop an interesting approach that incorporates priors (or uncertainties) on inputs but is still forced to make Gaussian assumptions to get good performance.

An entirely different approach is to make the decision about how significant each new configuration is using a stacked predictor. Each known set of values of the indicators, that is each observed point in the configuration space, is treated as a row of a dataset, and labelled according to whether it is significant or not. A data-analytic predictor is trained on this dataset usng any high-performing predictor (random forests, gradient boosted trees, support vector machines, or neural networks (Zaki and Meira 2020)). Each new configuration of indicators can then be fed to the predictor which outputs its prediction of whether or not it is significant.

Most high-performing predictors are black boxes – they make a prediction but do not explain why they made it. This can make it difficult to act on, since humans are more comfortable acting when they understand the justification for it. There are ways to elicit some of the reasons behind a particular prediction, but they are limited, especially when the number of indicators is large (Rozemberczki et al. 2022).

Hierarchical Models

So far, we have implicitly assumed a single monolithic set of indicators and a single decision of when a configuration is significant and requires action. However, many systems are hierarchically structured in some way, and responses specialised to some parts of the system may also be important. For example, a health emergency may take place in a geographically limited region, and a warning should be raised for that region, even though the emergency might not appear significant on a national or international scale. In a drug trial, the number of patients with side effects may be small overall, but the distribution of side effects within subpopulations must also be considered. In such settings, decisions about significance must happen at multiple scales, and so models must be hierarchically composable into larger models. It is also often the case that a large-scale adverse event is the result of a cascade of smaller ones. Appropriate detection and response to smaller adverse events might often have prevented a larger one (Ferguson 2021).

It is therefore prudent to design health intelligence warning systems in a hierarchical way. This does not substantially change the techniques needed; indeed, it can help by reducing the problems of scaling. There are some subtleties to consider: suppose that a particular indicator is an input to multiple lower-level systems, and the outputs of all of these systems are then inputs to a higher-level system. That indicator is, in a way, double counted in the higher-level system and may cause distortions as a result.

Conclusions

Health intelligence systems today are almost all based on collecting natural language reports from online sources, extracting counts of mentions of a range of diseases and syndromes, and presenting these, usually graphically, to human analysts. There are two drawbacks to such systems. First, online mentions of diseases or syndromes tend to occur only when they are unexpected. So, for example, there are very few mentions of ILI during flu season since its presence is entirely expected, Second, human analysts have to learn to make judgements about when the number of mentions requires action and it may take time and skill to make these judgements.

Developments in data analytics could straightforwardly provide new functionality in three ways. First, such systems can learn the temporal properties of disease and syndrome occurrences and so can derive thresholds for each regardless of the number of diseases or syndromes being considered. Second, they can use linear configuration spaces to detect when a constellation of diseases or syndromes is unusual, even if each independently is not. Third, they can use other forms of data such as counts derived directly from emergency room or physician visits, drug prescription data, vaccination rates and so on. Human analysts would still be needed but they would be presented with a more holistic, situational view.

Further enhancing health intelligence systems is more challenging, and a topic of active research. On the front end of the process, more research is needed on how to select good indicators (and then convincing governments to pay for their collection). As we have discussed, there are many open technical questions: how to incorporate Bayesian ideas into indicators, how to design richer configuration spaces, particularly nonlinear ones, and how to improve anomaly detection algorithms. Research is also needed on how best to present the situational awareness derived from configuration spaces to public health professionals, government and media.

COVID-19 has shown the importance of health intelligence systems, and developments in data analytics have shown how some of the challenges that health intelligence creates might be tackled computationally. There is a pressing need to make significant progress in this area if we have learned anything from the recent pandemic.

References

Alvarez, E., Bielska, I.A., Hopkins, S., et al. (2023). Limitations of COVID-19 testing and case data for evidence-informed health policy and practice. *Health Research Policy System*, 21: 11. https://doi.org/10.1186/s12961-023-00963-1

Andrews, R., Tickle, A.B., and Diederich, J. (2001). A review of techniques for extracting rules from trained artificial neural networks. *Clinical Applications of Artificial Neural Networks*, 256–297.

Andrews, S., Brewster, B., and Day, T. (2018). Organised crime and social media: A system for detecting, corroborating and visualising weak indicators of organised crime online. *Security Informatics*, 7: 3–20.

Ansoff, H.I. (1975). Managing strategic surprise by response to weak signals. *California Management Review*, XVIII(2): 21–33.

Arvanitidis, G., Hauberg, S., and Schölkopf, B. (2012). Geometrically enriched latent spaces. Proceedings of the 24th International Conference on Artificial Intelligence and Statistics. *PMLR*, 130: 631–639.

Beardsley, N.L. and Beech, A. (2013). Applying the Violent Extremist Risk Assessment (VERA) to a sample of terrorist case studies. *Journal of Aggression*, 5(1): 4–15.

Brynielsson, J., Horndahl, A., Johansson, F., Kaati, L., Mårtenson, C., and Svenson, P. (2013). Harvesting and analysis of weak indicators for detecting lone wolf terrorists. *Security Informatics*, 2: 11.

Dudenhoefer, A.-L., Niesse, C., Gorgen, T., Tampe, L., Megler, M., Gropler, C., and Bondü, R. (2021). Leaking in terrorist attacks: A review. *Aggression and Violent Behavior*, 58: 1359–1789.

Ferguson, N. (2021). *Doom*. Penguin Random House.

Holopainen, M. and Toivonen, M. (2012). Weak indicators: Ansoff today. *Futures*, 44, 198–205.

Hwang, Y.S. and Bang, S.Y. (1997). An efficient method to construct a radial basis function neural network classifier. *Neural Networks*, 10(8): 1495–1503.

Kajava, J., Savola, R., and Varonen, R. (2005). Weak indicators in information security management. International Conference on Computational and Information Science. CIS 2005: *Computational Intelligence and Security*, 508–517.

Kima, J. and Lee, C. (2017). Novelty-focused weak indicator detection in futuristic data: Assessing the rarity and paradigm unrelatedness of indicators. *Technological Forecasting & Social Change*, 120: 59–76.

Kingma, D.P. and Welling, M. (2019). An introduction to variational autoencoders. *Foundations and Trends in Machine Learning*, 12(4): 307–392.

Koivisto, R., Kulmala, I., and Gotcheva, N. (2016). Weak indicators and damage scenarios — Systematics to identify weak indicators and their sources related to mass transport attacks. *Technological Forecasting & Social Change*, 104: 180–190.

Lammers, J., Crusius, J., and Gasta, A. (2020). Correcting misperceptions of exponential coronavirus growth increases support for social distancing. *PNAS*, 117(28): 16264–17162.

MacIntyre, C.R., Chen, X., Kunasekaran, M., Quigley, Lim, A.S., Stone, H., Paik, H-Y., Yao, L., Heslop, D., Wei, W., Sarmiento, I. and Gurdasani, D. (2023). Artificial intelligence in public health: the potential of epidemic early warning systems. *Journal of International Medical Research*, 51(3):1–18.

Macrae, C. (2014). Early warnings, weak indicators and learning from healthcare disasters. *BMJ Quality Safety*, 23: 440–445.

Ojala, J. and Uskali, T. (2006). Any weak indicators? The New York Times and the stock market crashes of 1929, 1987 and 2000. XIV International Economic History Congress, Helsinki, p. 24.

Paltrinieri, N. and Khan, F. (eds.) (2016). *Dynamic Risk Analysis in the Chemical and Petroleum Industry, Evolution and Interaction with Parallel Disciplines in the Perspective of Industrial Application.* Butterworth Heinemann, Elsevier.

Papachristos, A.V. (2009). Murder by structure: Dominance relations and the social structure of gang homicide. *American Journal of Sociology*, 115: 74–128.

Pasman, H.J. (2020). Early warning indicators noticed, but management doesn't act adequately or not at all: A brief analysis and direction of possible improvement. *Journal of Loss Prevention Processing Induction Separation*, 9(4): 104272.

Phillips, P.J. and Pohl, G. (2020). How terrorism red flags become weak indicators through the processes of judgement and evaluation. *Journal of Police and Criminal Psychology*, 35: 377–388.

Roberts, E., Bassett, B.A., and Lochner, M. (2022). Bayesian Anomaly Detection and Classification. arXiv:1902.08627. https://arxiv.org/abs/1902.08627

Rozemberczki, B., Watson, L., Bayer, P., Yang, H.-T., Kiss, O., Nilsson, S., and Sarkar, R. The Shapley Value in Machine Learning. arXiv 2202.05594. https://arxiv.org/abs/2202.05594

Schoemaker, P.J.H. and Day, G.S. (2009). How to make sense of weak indicators. *MIT SLOAN Management Review*, 50(3): 81–89.

Scientific American (2022). U.S. Monkeypox Response Has Been Woefully Inadequate, Experts Say. www.scientificamerican.com/article/monkeypox-testing-and-vaccination-in-u-s-have-been-vastly-inadequate-experts-say1/

Skillicorn, D.B. (2007). *Understanding Complex Datasets: Matrix Decompositions for Data Mining.* Volume I of the Chapman & Hall/CRC Data Mining and Knowledge Discovery Series.

Skillicorn, D.B. (2012). Outlier detection using semantic sensors. 2012 IEEE International Conference on Intelligence and Security Informatics. IEEE.

Sornette, D. and Ouillon, G. (2012). Dragon-kings: Mechanisms, statistical methods and empirical evidence. *The European Physical Journal Special Topics*, 205(1): 1–26.

Taleb, N. (2010). *The Black Swan: The Impact of the Highly Improbable*, 2nd ed. Random House Publishing Group.

van der Maaten, L. and Hinton, G. (2008). Visualizing data using t-SNE. *Journal of Machine Learning Research*, 9: 11.

Veerman, J.L., Mackenbach, J.P., and Barendregt, J.J. (2007). Validity of predictions in health impact assessment. *Journal of Epidemiology Community Health*, 61(4): 362–366.

Vogt, S. (2017). Innovation in European Police Forces. *European Police Science and Research Bulletin*, 4: 283–286.

von Luxburg, U. (2007). A tutorial on spectral clustering. *Statistics and Computing*, 17: 395–416.

Wucker, M. (2016). *The Gray Rhino: How to Recognize and Act on the Obvious Dangers We Ignore*. St Martins Press.

Zaki, M.J. and Meira, Jr., W. (2020). *Data Mining and Machine Learning: Fundamental Concepts and Algorithms*, 2nd ed. Cambridge University Press. https://dataminingbook.info/

7 Biosecurity, National Security Intelligence and Ethics

Seumas Miller

Introduction

The focus of this chapter is on various ethical issues that arise at the interface of biosecurity problems (construed as a subset of what are often referred to as health security issues) and national security intelligence activity (Miller 2009: Ch. 7; MacLeish 2017; Walsh 2018; Davis 2021; Walsh 2021). Needless to say, there are many biosecurity problems that do not constitute national security problems and there are many national security problems that have nothing to do with biosecurity. Our interest is with biosecurity problems that *do* constitute national security problems (at least potentially) and that, therefore, require national security intelligence activity. More specifically, our interest is with the ethical dimension of such national security intelligence (NSI) activity.

Prior to discussing the national security problems addressed in this chapter we need to get some clarity on the concepts of biosecurity, biosafety and national security (discussed in the first section), and on the relation between individual rights, security and collective goods explored in this chapter. In doing so we acknowledge that definitions of all these concepts are somewhat vague, contestable and that therefore a degree of stipulation is inevitable. (For somewhat different definitions from those offered here, see Dahl 2024, and Walsh et al. 2023, in this volume and Walsh 2018, 10–13.) The national security ethical issues addressed thereafter arise in the following contexts: Biobank and Database Security, and NSI and Bulk Databases (third section); Pandemics (fourth section) and; Dual Use Problems (fifth section).

Biosecurity, Biosafety and National Security

In what follows we must distinguish between security and safety and, therefore, between biosecurity and biosafety, notwithstanding the close relationship between these two concepts.

On our account security presupposes a malevolent individual or organisation possessed of an *intention* to do harm, whereas safety does not presuppose such an intention. Thus, accidental harm is a safety issue whereas intended harm is a security issue. We note, however, a grey area, namely, culpable negligence.

DOI: 10.4324/9781003335511-10

Arguably, culpable negligence should be regarded as a security issue, notwithstanding the absence of an intention to do harm (Miller 2018, 9). Consider the COVID-19 pandemic. While the debate on the initial cause of the outbreak of COVID-9 in China continues to rage, it may be the case, firstly, that SARS-CoV-2 escaped from a Wuhan laboratory in China resulting eventually in the COVID-19 pandemic and, secondly, that the escape resulted from lax, indeed culpable, biocontainment (Rabinowitz 2023). If so, then the initial escape was a biosecurity beach and not merely a biosafety breach. Of course, ultimately, COVID-19 became a major biosafety and biosecurity issue. If a person is infected, then they are a risk to others. If this person is asymptomatic, does not know that they are infected, and reasonably could not know this, then they constitute a biosafety risk but not necessarily a biosecurity risk (although they might ultimately become a biosecurity risk). If they do know that they are infected yet refuse to take reasonable steps to avoid contact with other persons, then they constitute a biosecurity risk. More generally, a pandemic is a biosecurity issue, as opposed to a biosafety issue, insofar as members of a population are aware that, if infected, they pose a potential threat to the lives of themselves and others, which they can choose to minimise (e.g., by complying with symptom monitoring, testing, contact tracing and tracking, quarantine requirements, hand washing, social distancing, mask wearing, and, ultimately, vaccination (Miller and Smith 2021; Miller and Smith 2023; Sorell 2023). While the danger emanates from the transmissible, virulent pathogen, nevertheless, it is the irresponsible behaviour of human beings that transforms this safety issue into a security issue.

Thus, by the lights of our distinction between biosafety and biosecurity, the COVID-19 pandemic involved both biosafety and biosecurity issues. At any rate, in this chapter we will treat culpable negligence as a security issue rather than merely a safety issue.

Accordingly, if an adversary designs, manufactures and/or uses bioweapons this is clearly a biosecurity issue. If the bioweapon is in the hands of terrorist groups it is a bioterrorism issue (and potentially also a biowarfare issue depending on the nature and scale of the threat it poses, e.g., a few anthrax letters sent to terrorise public officials, as in Amerithrax (CCR 2002), would not constitute biowarfare). If the bioweapon is in the hands of state actors it is a biowarfare issue (and potentially also a bioterrorism issue depending on whether the civilians are targets but also on whether using bioweapons against combatants is deemed to be terrorism). On the other hand, if an unpredictable earthquake causes the collapse of a building in which there is an otherwise properly designed and maintained laboratory containing hazardous biological material then the consequence of this natural disaster is a biosafety issue, supposing there is now a high risk of exposure to this material. Now consider gain of function (GOF) research conducted on a pathogen to enhance its transmissibility (Selgelid 2016). An instance of GOF research was the so-called ferret flu experiments conducted on the deadly flu virus H5N1 by scientists in the US and the Netherlands. While H5NI causes bird flu it could cross species barriers and infect humans. Accordingly, these experiments were designated experiments of concern and constituted dual use experiments (NSABB 2015; Miller and Selgelid

2007; van der Bruggen et al. 2011; Miller 2013; Miller 2018, 12–14). We discuss these issues further in the fifth section below on dual use problems. Here we simply note that if the enhanced pathogen were to escape from the laboratory due to culpable negligence with respect to biocontainment requirements, then this would be a biosecurity issue – at least on our account of the distinction between biosafety and biosecurity.

It might be thought that the conceptual distinction between safety and security and, therefore, between biosafety and biosecurity while it is interesting from a theoretical perspective, nevertheless, does not have great practical significance. However, on the contrary, the distinction has considerable institutional and, therefore, practical significance. Obviously, the remit of national security agencies, including NSI agencies, is national security. By contrast, there are an array of other institutions that have responsibilities in respect of various forms of safety, including the safety of drugs and food (e.g., the US Food and Drug Administration), sewage health and safety (e.g., Water Quality Australia), safety of buildings and bridges (e.g., Bridge Health and Safety (UK)), bushfire (wildfire) safety (e.g., rural fire brigades), disaster prevention and relief (e.g., tsunami and earthquake warning systems, disaster relief agencies), and the protection of coral reef eco-systems (e.g., the Australian Reef Authority is responsible for the Great Barrier Reef).

Let us set aside the question as to whether it would be an efficient and effective use of resources to widen the remit of national security agencies so that it included dealing with safety issues, although it is surely self-evident that such a radical program of institutional redesign would not be rational in terms of the division of institutional labour in a complex modern nation-state. The point to be stressed here is that given the intrusive powers of NSI agencies and, inter alia, their requirements to collect (often on a large-scale) and analyse sensitive personal and confidential data, it would be highly morally problematic for a liberal democracy to extend the remit of its national security agencies, and NSI agencies in particular, in this manner. Of course, as mentioned above in relation to pandemics, many natural disasters and other safety issues are also, or ultimately give rise to, security issues, including national security issues. Accordingly, there is a need at times for NSI agencies and those institutions responsible for various forms of safety to collaborate. Thus, national security agencies might benefit from detailed information provided by detection and early warning systems in relation to pandemics, given the potential for the emergence of national security problems. This collaboration might involve inter alia NSI agencies getting access to personal or confidential information that they might not otherwise be entitled to. For instance, they might get access to sensitive health and smartphone information; information used to determine a person's health, whereabouts and movements for contact tracing and tracking in order to identify potentially infected individuals in the context of combatting a pandemic. However, such access might have the potential via 'mission creep' to enable the security agencies to create or enhance movement profiles and, thereby, violate privacy rights.

The notion of security is vague, contested and used to refer to various form of security, notably various forms of collective security. The forms of collective security include the traditional ones of national security and community security. An instance of a current grave threat to national security, and the national security of Ukraine in particular, is the current ongoing Russian invasion of that country. An instance of a current threat to the security of a community is the recent well-publicised dramatic increase in alcohol-fuelled assaults, shop break-ins, car burnings and other crimes perpetrated by indigenous youths in the town of Alice Springs in Central Australia which has evidently spread fear in the local community, resulted in a curfew being imposed and undermined community security (Cassidy 2024). Here, as elsewhere, the long-term solution might not lie principally in the response of the security agencies, i.e., the police, but rather in addressing the underlying socio-economic and other conditions; when dealing with security problems, prevention is better than cure. At any rate, our concern is with biosecurity which, of course, can be a matter of community security and/or of national security. Thus, the Soviet bioweapons program created a biosecurity risk for its adversary nation-states and their communities (Shoham and Wolfson 2004). Again, community security problems can escalate to the point at which they become national security problems, as seems to have happened in Haiti where violent gangs have taken over most of the capital city, Port-au-Prince (Coto 2024). It follows that these various forms of collective security are not mutually exclusive. Moreover, there is a further point to be made here. Biosecurity problems can also give rise to *global* security problems; problems confronting, as it were, the entire 'community' of nation-states and their populations. Thus, bioweapons constitute a biosecurity problem and, as a consequence, a community and a national security problem. However, since bioweapons are typically in the hands of the security agencies of adversary nation-states (and, potentially, in the hands of terrorist groups with transnational agendas) they also constitute a global security problem. Pandemics are another instance of a potential global security problem. Indeed, the COVID-19 pandemic constituted a global biosafety problem and, arguably, also a global biosecurity problem. We return to this issue in the fourth section on pandemics below.

As we saw above, in relation to the conceptual distinction between safety and security, it might be thought that the conceptual distinction between national security and other forms of collective security, and that between biosecurity threats that rise to the level of national security and ones that do not, while interesting from a theoretical perspective do not have great practical significance. However, by parity of reasoning with respect to the safety/security distinction, these distinctions in respect of national security also have considerable institutional and, therefore, practical significance. At the risk of restating the obvious, by contrast with national security agencies, including NSI agencies, there are an array of institutions that have responsibilities in respect of various forms of security other than national security. These include local police services concerned with crime and community security in their jurisdiction, private security firms that protect homes or businesses, multiple private and public sector cybersecurity incident response teams, corporate fraud and corruption units, and so on. As above, let us set aside the question as to whether it would be an efficient and effective use of resources to widen the remit of national security agencies so that it included dealing with all or most of these security issues (although self-evidently it would not be rational for a complex modern nation-state to do so). The point to be stressed here is essentially the one made above in relation to institutions responsible for various forms of safety, namely, that given the intrusive powers of NSI agencies it would be highly morally problematic for a liberal democracy to extend their remit in this manner, given that in a liberal democracy domestic police organisations, private security organisations and the like are justifiably constrained in their intelligence activities to a greater extent than NSI agencies are. Indeed, there have already been concerns in relation to, for instance, counter-terrorism that NSI agencies in the US and elsewhere have engaged in overreach (and, at times, unlawful overreach) and, thereby, arguably violated the privacy and other moral rights of their citizens (e.g., the US National Security Agency (NSA) bulk data collection of the metadata of US citizens (Walsh and Miller 2016)).

The Moral Right to Individual Security, National Security and Collective Goods

Thus far we have distinguished biosecurity from biosafety, and national security from other forms of collective security. However, there are, of course, a variety of forms of individual security, as opposed to collective security, relevant to biosecurity; notably personal physical security. Personal physical security pertains to (justified or unjustified) threats to one's life (e.g., the use of bioweapons), physical movement (e.g., curfews) or physical wellbeing (e.g., an infected person knowingly spreading a disease).

The notion of physical security embraces not only threats to personal physical security but also threats to inanimate objects such as buildings, physical property and the like, although the biological threats to inanimate objects are likely to be indirect, (e.g., as a result of anti-lockdown protests in a pandemic). Moreover, the physical things that we seek at times to secure, whether they be animate or inanimate, are not necessarily goods, such as life, freedom and property. For we seek to secure, or at least, safely contain, harmful or dangerous things, such as toxins, pathogens and infected humans (e.g., by means of quarantine). By the lights of our account of the distinction between safety and security, security (but not safety) presupposes the actuality or possibility of: (i) an external intentional attack or threat of an intentional attack (e.g., the Soviet bioweapons program, the WannaCry ransomware attack in 2017 on the UK National Health Service (Collier 2017); (ii) an internal intentional breach of a protective system (e.g., unauthorised disclosure of confidential information as in the case of Edward Snowden's leaking of classified documents (Walsh and Miller 2016) and, in the case of Abdul Qadeer Khan, his 1976 theft from the Anglo-Dutch-German nuclear engineering consortium, Urenco, of classified scientific information which made a crucial contribution to Pakistan nuclear weapons programme (Albright and Hinderstein 2004)); or (iii) culpable negligence on the part of an internal or external actor (e.g., the above-mentioned *alleged* escape from a Wuhan laboratory of SARS-CoV-2 as a result of lax biocontainment, and the 1984 Bhopal toxic gas disaster which caused thousands of deaths, and hundreds of thousands of injuries, and resulted in the conviction of a number of employees for culpable negligence (Cassels 1991)).

The notion of security in so far as it pertains directly or indirectly to human beings (our concern in this chapter), embraces not only physical security but also psychological, institutional and of particular interest to us in the third section below, data security. Psychological security is a form of individual security whereas institutional security is a form of collective security. Harassment on social media may threaten one's psychological security; Russian interference in the 2016 US Presidential elections constituted a threat to US democratic institutions (Mueller 2019). By contrast, data security might be a form of individual security (e.g., if an individual's sensitive medical data is stolen) or a form of institutional security (e.g., if a NSI agency's secret intelligence is stolen).

An important distinction to be made here is that between the security of those things or features to which one has moral rights and those things or features to which one does not have a moral right. One has moral rights to one's life, freedom, privacy, physical property, personal data and so on but not (at least typically) to *someone's else's* life, freedom, privacy, physical property or personal data. However, the concept of security can apply not only to things or features to which one has a moral right but also to things or features to which one does *not* have a moral right. Thus, a thief might secure property he stole to prevent its being retrieved by the person he stole it from. He might have a security problem with respect to this property, but he does not have a security *right* in respect of it; it does not belong to him. In short, security per se is not necessarily a moral right; it all depends on whether one has a moral right to the thing or feature being secured.

Since most, perhaps all, moral rights are not absolute and, therefore, can under certain circumstances justifiably be overridden, then the associated security rights can typically also justifiably be overridden. Thus, one's right to personal data and, therefore, to the security of that data in, for instance, a genomic database such as Ancestry.com, can be overridden under certain circumstances, such as by law enforcement officers investigating a murder and needing to access a suspect's DNA data held in the Ancestry.com database (Smith 2018; Smith and Miller 2021, 39–54; Miller and Smith 2022). Now consider the accessing of personal data in the context of a pandemic such as COVID-19. Metadata might help to identify individuals who need to be tested for COVID-19 because they may have been in close contact with an infected person. Moreover, this need may well override the privacy right to one's metadata (Miller and Smith 2023).

Personal (physical) security is a more fundamental notion than collective security. Indeed, collective security in its various forms is in large part derived from personal security. Thus COVID-19, for example, is a threat to public health and national security precisely because it threatens the lives and physical well-being of individual citizens. However, collective security is not simply aggregate personal (physical) security. For example, COVID-19 might be a threat to the integrity of *institutions*, including public health institutions.

Notions of collective security, national security, global security and so on are collective goods. There is evidently a family resemblance between notions such as *common good, collective good, common interest, collective interest, public good, public interest* and so on. Such goods or interests are attached to, or are enjoyed by, groups and other collectives, such as the collective good of Australian people (e.g., public health) or the collective interest of the pharmaceutical industry (e.g., record profits). The contrast here is between common goods, common interests (or, in our parlance, collective goods), on the one hand, and a single person's interest or a benefit that is or could be produced and/or enjoyed by a single person. Historically, notions of the common good, collective interest and the like in the political sphere are associated with philosophers such as Aristotle, Aquinas, Hobbes and Rousseau. Here we need to draw attention to the possibility of collective goods and collective interests in which the collective in question is the world's population; that is, we need to note the existence of global collective goods and global collective interests. The threat posed by climate change to the world's population is one instance; the world's population has a collective interest in combating climate change. Another instance is the collective interest of the world's population in avoiding pandemics.

There is a distinction to be made between the collective good in general and specific collective goods. Security, public health and an efficient transport system are all examples of specific collective goods. We can presumably, at least in principle, draw up a list of such specific collective goods. In what follows we shall focus on what we are referring to as collective goods and put some restrictions on the meaning of that term. Collective goods in our favoured sense (Miller 2001, 217–220; Miller 2010, 66–76) are goods that are produced, maintained or renewed by collective action. Moreover, members of a community or citizens of a nation-state may have a collective moral responsibility to produce, maintain or renew certain collective goods, e.g., national security, and in order to do so they have a collective responsibility (Miller 2001: Ch. 8; Miller 2010, Ch. 4) to perform the collective actions that are the means to realise the collective goods in question. In complex modern societies these collective responsibilities are typically discharged in large part by members of institutions; institutions that have as their raison d'etre or institutional purpose to produce or maintain the relevant collective goods (Miller 2010). Naturally, particular institutions, such as military forces and NSI agencies, have been established to maintain the collective good of national security. However, in times of war, for instance, maintaining this collective good requires the contribution of virtually the whole citizenry and not simply the members of the military forces and of NSI agencies. In time of war there is a collective moral responsibility on the part of all, or most, citizens to contribute to the war effort. Likewise, in relation to pandemics the collective good of public health and, relatedly, security, requires the contribution of virtually the whole citizenry and not simply the members of the public health institutions and relevant security agencies, e.g., police to enforce quarantine restrictions, NSI agencies to identify the threat of a pandemic to enable adequate preparations (Feltes 2021; Miller and Smith 2023).

National security is a good by virtue of the thing secured, namely the nation, specifically the liberal democratic nation-state, being a good (a collective good). Ultimately, the liberal democratic nation-state is itself a collective good, indeed a collective *moral* good, in so far as it embodies, respects and protects the moral rights of the members of its population. NSI activity is, therefore, in the service of a collective good which is a moral good, namely, national security. Moreover, national security activity on the part members of NSI agencies is a moral responsibility, a collective moral responsibility. This collective moral responsibility is derivable from the collective moral good of national security (Miller 2022).

It is important to distinguish between national security and national interest (and between both of these concepts and what might be thought to be, or presented as, national security or national interest, respectively). Clearly, all manner of autocrats and demagogues (especially) have falsely claimed that some policy which is really only in their own political interest, or only in the interest of their political party, is in fact in the national interest; or is a matter of national security. So it is important to determine what is, objectively speaking, in the national interest. It is also important to determine what is, again objectively speaking, a matter of national security. However, it is also important to distinguish the concept of national security from the concept of national interest although, of course, it is in the national interest to preserve national security. However, national interest is a much wider notion than national security. The remit of national security agencies does not, or ought not, include acting in the national interest on matters that are not matters of national security.

That said, the content of the term 'national security' is notoriously ill-defined, indeterminate, open-ended and contestable. Moreover, the concepts of national security and national interest can be conflated. Importantly, national security should not simply be understood as national interest since the latter notion is very permissive and could license all manner of individual and collective rights violations. For instance, it might be in the national interest of a nation state to increase its territory by invading a neighbouring nation state. Perhaps the Russian invasion of Ukraine might ultimately be thought to have been in Russia's national interest, assuming that Russia ends up acquiring not only Crimea but also, say, the Donbas industrial region of eastern Ukraine. Again, it might be thought to be in the national interest of some nation states to enslave a population, or to otherwise engage in widespread, serious rights' violations, to increase its own wealth. Historically, the slave trade was thought to be an economic imperative and, therefore, in the interest of, for instance, the US during the eighteenth century. The Chinese incarceration of hundreds of thousands of Uighurs in oil and resources-rich Xinjiang might be thought by members of the Chinese communist party to be in the national interest.

However, as noted above, national security is not the same concept as national interest. National security involves serious internal or external (direct or indirect) threats to the nation state itself, or to one of its fundamental political, military, criminal justice or economic institutions, and that these threats might emanate from state or non-state actors, such as terrorist groups. NSI pertains to such threats. So NSI includes military intelligence, but also some criminal intelligence and economic intelligence, since the latter may have national security implications. Consider, for instance, intelligence on drug cartels destabilising governments or on fighter aircraft being built by private companies. Note also that while national security threats (as opposed to safety threats) are necessarily posed by state or non-state (and, therefore, human) actors, the conditions under which these security threats emerge might have arisen as a result of other, including non-human, sources, such as (at least in some cases) pandemics, famines or water shortages consequent on climate change.

A final point regarding collective or common goods. Economists typically speak of a species of common goods that are *public* goods. They define public goods as being nonrival and nonexcludable. If a good is nonrival, then my enjoyment of it does not prevent or diminish the possibility of your enjoyment of it (e.g., a street sign is nonrival since my using it to find my way has no effect on you likewise using it). Again, a nonexcludable good means that, if anyone is enjoying it, then no one can be prevented from enjoying it (e.g., national security). The public goods in question are typically relativised to the nation-state but increasingly to the global economy. Non-rivalness and non-excludability are relevant to the characterisation of collective goods. However, the notion of a collective good is not necessarily defined in terms of them. Other properties relevant to the notion of a collective good include jointness of production. Collective goods in our sense are jointly produced, maintained or renewed. And perhaps, if a collective good is enjoyed, then it is enjoyed by all; or if not, it ought to be. However, the point not to be stressed here is that collective goods in our sense might or might not be public goods in the economists' sense.

Biobank and Database Security

Data in, or extracted from, biobanks and health, medical, biometric and human genomic databases (NHGRI 2019) is increasing and the technology to analyse it is becoming more sophisticated (e.g., AI technology). Much of this data and the results of it are potentially available to law enforcement, including NSI, agencies, e.g., to enable their pandemic threat assessments. The recent COVID-19 pandemic has given impetus to this process (Davis 2021; Macnish and Henschke 2023). Moreover, forensic biometric databases (e.g., fingerprint databases) and genomic databases (e.g., DNA databases) are larger and more reliable, given recent developments in science and technology (Smith 2018; Smith and Miller 2021; Miller and Smith 2022). In so far as these developments facilitate legitimate NSI purposes they are welcome. However, there are actual and potential moral costs in terms of privacy and confidentiality, and specifically in terms of data security broadly construed. For health, medical, biometric and genomic databanks are vulnerable to inter alia cyberattacks, thereby potentially threatening critical infrastructure (Miller and Bossomaier 2024: Ch. 5). Moreover, the vulnerability of forensic databanks gives rise, in some instances, to additional national security risks – additional to the ones the data in some of these databanks was being used to address, (e.g., successful cyberattacks on forensic DNA databases compromising criminal cases, including national security criminal cases).

In this section our concern is with the ethical issues that arise in the context of threats to the data security of biobanks and health, medical, biometric and genomic (including forensic) databases, and especially what is morally at stake in respect of this data security. What is morally at stake turns in part on what moral rights there are to the data under threat of, say, theft or destruction, e.g., violation of privacy rights, and in part on what further harmful consequences might flow if data rights are violated, e.g., by ransomware attacks. It also turns on what collective goods result from the collection, storage and analysis of this data, e.g., public health, national security, as well as on what collective harms might potentially be done if it is collected in the first place, e.g., universal DNA databases arguably contribute to a power imbalance between the state and the citizenry (Miller and Smith 2022).

The terms 'biobank' and 'database' are often not well-defined. We will use the 'term' biobank to refer to a large, structured collection of human or non-human (e.g., plant, animal or microbe (including pathogens) biological material and related data or information. By contrast, we will use the term, 'database' to refer to large, structured collections of data or information which might or might not relate to biological material and might or might not also contain biological material. Moreover, the biobanks and databases of interest here are ones relevant to our biosecurity concerns; they are not necessarily restricted to ones that are only used for research. Thus, as mentioned above, DNA databases, for instance, are often used for forensic purposes by law enforcement agencies, including national security agencies, and may contain samples. However, we do need to keep in mind the distinction between forensic databases established for law enforcement and/ or NSI purposes and non-forensic biobanks and databases not held by security agencies but to which NSI agencies might have access (perhaps on a piecemeal basis under warrant).

Further, we distinguish between data and information; and between both of these concepts and knowledge. Data is not the same as information, let alone knowledge. Data can be false and in need of clarification, interpretation and verification. Moreover, if we assume that information is not only meaningful but also true, accurate, probable, or otherwise in some sense correct, information might, nevertheless, not constitute knowledge, since knowledge is typically regarded as a true, accurate, probable, correct belief, statement, report etc., for which one has good and decisive evidence (Miller 2022). Because data is not the same as information, let alone knowledge, whether the data is ultimately useful depends on the capacity to clarify, verify and adequately interpret the raw data and such interpretation involves inter alia setting the data in question in a pre-existing framework of knowledge, e.g., within the framework of pre-existing knowledge (or, at least, presumed knowledge) of the human genome; consequently, accessing data in and of itself may not provide meaningful information, let alone useful knowledge. Moreover, if health, medical, biometric, genomic and other data, information or knowledge, or the results of the analysis of same, constitutes national security intelligence, and is thus relevant to NSI agencies, then it needs to be actionable; the intelligence products of NSI agencies must be actionable, including by virtue of being disseminated to, and adequately grasped by, the NSI agencies' political masters.

As we have seen, biobanks, health, genomic and other bulk databases are typically the means to provide collective goods, such as public health (e.g., databases of those infected by communicable diseases and biobanks used to conduct research and develop vaccines), and security (e.g. forensic DNA databases) or both (e.g., pandemic surveillance databases). Moreover, as we have also seen, in some instances individuals have collective moral responsibilities to provide the samples or data to enable the construction of these collections.

The notion of collective responsibility in play here is connected to the prior notion of a joint or cooperative action. Roughly speaking, a joint action can be understood thus: two or more individual persons perform a joint action if each of them intentionally performs his or her action but does so with the (true) belief that, in so doing each will do their part, and they will jointly realise an end that each of them has, and which each has interdependently with the others (i.e., a collective end) (Miller 2001, Ch. 8; Miller 2010, Ch. 4; Miller and Feltes 2021; Feltes 2021). On this view collective responsibility is joint responsibility and, therefore, collective responsibility is ascribed to individuals. Moreover, if the joint action in question is morally significant (e.g., by virtue of the collective end being a collective good or a collective harm), then other things being equal the individuals are collectively *morally* responsible for it. Each member of the group is individually responsible for his or her own contributory action and, at least in the case of most small-scale joint action, each is also individually (fully or partially) responsible for the aimed at outcome (i.e., the realised collective end) of the joint action. However, each is individually responsible for the realised collective end, *jointly with the others*. Hence, the conception is relational in character. Moreover, if the collective end of the joint action is a collective good or a collective harm, then these individual persons are collectively morally responsible for this good or harm.

In the case of bulk databases, the joint action called for is joint *epistemic* action (from the ancient Greek work, 'episteme', meaning knowledge); each individual is providing some information rather than performing a behavioural action and, of course, there are a very large number of individuals contributing their data (Miller 2022). However, in general the data or information, if it is health or medical data, requires their consent to be collected since it is data to which they have some sort of prior moral (and frequently legal) control right, e.g., it is governed by their right to privacy.

Many large-scale, health and medical data collection, storage and analysis facilities are referred to as health and medical information commons (HMIC). Roughly speaking, it is a commons by virtue of two main properties: (1) the personal data in question is provided by a large number of the members of whole populations (i.e., the aggregated data is jointly provided); (2) the aggregated data constitutes a structured knowledge base of big data (a collective epistemic entity) that, since it is ultimately in the service of a collective good such as public health (e.g., via the use of data analytics), is itself an instrumental good (i.e., an epistemic collective good). However, there are numerous other bulk databases which provide collective epistemic goods and which directly or indirectly can assist

NSI activity. These include law enforcement and NSI databases of offenders and their offences, fingerprints, DNA, photos, associates, intelligence reports and so on but also numerous other public and private sector databases of names, phone numbers, email addresses, social media accounts, social security accounts, facial images scraped from the internet, car number plates, bank accounts, credit card numbers, tax files and so on. All of these databases are, at least in principle, potentially accessible to NSI agencies, even if in liberal democracies in many cases only under warrant. Moreover, there is the technical possibility to integrate these databases and to link persons, accounts and so on (via integration platforms such as Palantir used in the private sector). Further, there is the technical possibility of integrating these databases with surveillance technology, such as CCTV and facial recognition technology. China's social credit system is demonstrating just what can be achieved in this area; China appears to be on the way to establishing what amounts to a so-called surveillance state. One way to think of such a state is as one confronting a major national security threat to the citizenry but a threat emanating from the national security agencies of the state – the institutions whose responsibility is to protect the citizenry from national security threats. In short national security agencies, including NSI agencies, provide the collective good of national security but they also have the potential to threaten it if left to operate without constraints.

The constraints in question include institutional purpose, i.e., the collective good of national security (Miller 2022), and the principles of discrimination ('do not target the innocent'), necessity and proportionality (Miller 2021; Henschke et al. 2024). Accordingly, in determining whether or not it is morally and legally permissible for NSI agencies to establish any given bulk database (e.g., a universal DNA database), or to have some right of access to an existing bulk database not held in a NSI agency or other law enforcement agency (e.g., health, medical, biometric and genomic databases held in a wide array of public and private sector organisations), there needs to be recourse to considerations of institutional purpose and to the principles of necessity, proportionality and discrimination. Moreover, in order to ensure accountability, NSI agency access to external databases might require a warrant issued by a judicial officer in accordance with these principles.

There are individual rights to the data and to the collective goods, such as public health and, in the cases of interest to us, national security which itself may depend on the maintenance of public health, e.g., prevention of pandemics (see the fifth section below). However, matters are more complex than this, since there is an intervening collective *epistemic* good – namely the aggregated data. This collective good is epistemic since it consists in information or perhaps knowledge, and it is an instrumental good by virtue of being a means to realise the goods of public health and security. The question that now arises pertains to the nature of the ownership, or moral rights, to this collective epistemic good. After all, any data element pertaining to a single person is unimportant considered on its own. It is only the aggregate of data that has utility. Big data is the means to the end. We suggest that this collective epistemic good is jointly owned by those who contributed their personal data (Miller and Bossomaier 2024, Ch. 5).

Of what does this joint ownership consist, given that the data in question needs to be analysed if it is to be useful for public health and security purposes? Presumably, the joint owners of the data contribute their data on the condition that it is analysed in certain ways, to realise certain purposes (e.g., to prevent and mitigate diseases). However, it would not follow from this that their joint rights to the data and, for that matter, the underlying individual rights to it, had been extinguished.

Clearly the existence of biobanks or databases gives rise to data security concerns. Data security is compromised if unauthorised actors gain access to the biological material or data in question and either steal it (and potentially release it), tamper with it (or otherwise change it) or destroy it. In the case of human biometric, genomic, medical or healthcare data, unauthorised access may consist of the violation of one or more of the following related moral (and possibly legal) principles: privacy rights; confidentiality; autonomy rights (e.g., rights of an individual to control their data); personal identity rights (e.g., biometric data); ownership (e.g., intellectual property rights). We take that data pertaining to features of one's personal identity includes such things as DNA data and facial images (Miller and Bossomaier 2024, Ch. 5).

In the light of the above discussion, we can identify some of what is morally at stake when the data security of biobanks and health, medical, biometric and genomic databases is compromised. Self-evidently, one or more of the individual moral rights mentioned above, namely, privacy, autonomy and personal identity might have been violated; moreover, the moral principles of confidentiality and ownership might have been flouted. Further, if data security breaches become widespread then individuals might not provide their personal health, medical, biometric or genomic data, supposing this to be optional. Indeed, in some cases their collective moral responsibility to do so might be overridden or, at least, they might think it is, given the moral costs to themselves in terms of privacy and other violations, if they do. Consider, for instance, people who have self-tested positive for COVID but suffer only mild symptoms. They might be reluctant to provide their health data, including their test results, location and movements for the purposes of contact tracing and tracking, given they do not believe public health authorities are able to prevent data security breaches. This reluctance may undermine provision of the public health and national security benefits, i.e., the collective goods, of the databanks in question.

Aside from the failure to provide collective goods, there are the collective harms caused by some biobank or data security breaches. Depending on the nature and extent of these harms, they may have national security implications, as in the case of an attack on critical public health but also the possibility of samples of pathogens, such as Ebola, held in biobanks being stolen and used for bioterrorism. Moreover, if the data security of biometric and genomic databases, such as DNA databases, is compromised then this might directly impact national security institutions themselves, e.g., adversarial foreign states accessing DNA data in conjunction with open source and other information may be able to generate the genetic identity of, say, US field agents and other national security personnel (Rioss 2022, 1397). Finally, there is the threat posed by universal forensic databases, e.g., universal

DNA databases, and especially by the integration of these databases with a wide array of bulk databases, including (but not limited to) health, medical, biometric and genomic data established for research and health purposes. Here the spectre of the surveillance state, as is evident in the case of China's Uighur population in Xinjiang (Qiang 2019), looms large.

Pandemics

As noted above, pandemics are a potential security problem (as well as a safety problem). In the case of the COVID-19 pandemic, an actual serious security problem arose by very large numbers of people knowingly or, at least, negligently – i.e., by refusing to take reasonable precautions against its spread, such as by getting vaccinated; or, in the case of political leaders, refusing to implement policies enabling and requiring people to take reasonable precautions – infecting other people, leading to the severe illnesses and deaths of very large numbers of people, e.g. over one million in the US.

Inadequate regulation of cyberspace, and of social media platforms in particular, has enabled antivaxxers to spread disinformation, propaganda, and conspiracy theories in order to discredit vaccination programmes and, typically, play down the severity of the virus. This has had the effect of facilitating the spread of the pandemic by virtue of the large numbers of unvaccinated people who, nevertheless, continue to interact with others as though being infected was not a serious health risk. In some cases, antivaxxers have engaged in violent protests, like the so-called freedom convoy to Ottawa in early 2022, which led to the shutdown of the downtown area of a major city, the closure of a major US/Canada border crossing for a couple of weeks and the declaration of a state of emergency by the premier of Ontario (Woods and Pringle 2022).

Moreover, the problem has been compounded by foreign intervention and, specifically, the use of computational propaganda by Russia and China, in particular, in the overall national security context of the waging of cognitive warfare against Western liberal democracies (Miller 2023). Regarding computation propaganda, the advent of social media platforms and the associated cybertechnologies, such as algorithms and automated software (e.g. bots that mimic real people), has brought with it an exponential increase in the spread of disinformation, misinformation, conspiracy theories, hate speech and propaganda on the part of a wide array of actors, including individual citizens, single-issue pressure groups, right-wing and left-wing extremist groups, terrorist groups, criminal organisations, and, importantly in relation to our concerns here, state actors, notably Russia and China. Cognitive warfare is a recent development that makes use of computational propaganda. Cognitive warfare emerged from prior related non-kinetic forms of warfare, such as PsyOps operations and Information Warfare. In doing so it has relied heavily on new communication and information technologies, notably AI. Key features of cognitive warfare include its targeting of entire populations (as opposed to, for instance, merely military ones in wartime), its focus on changing a population's behaviour by way of changing its way of thinking rather than merely by the provision of discrete bits of false information in respect of specific issues (e.g., denying the extent of casualties in a kinetic war), its reliance on increasingly sophisticated psychological techniques of manipulation, and its aim of destabilising institutions, especially governments, albeit often indirectly by way of initially destabilising epistemic institutions, such as news media organisations and universities. Importantly, cognitive warfare has been able to harness the new channels of public communication, such as social media, upon which populations have become increasingly reliant. Moreover, in some contrast with traditional ideological contestation, e.g., the ideological conflict between the Soviet Union and the West during the Cold War, in which each of the protagonists have a system or quasi-system of ideas to try to 'sell', cognitive warfare also has a very strong initial focus on sowing division and undermining cooperation in its target population by emphasising existing differences and promoting polarising views, e.g., promoting both extreme left-wing *and* extreme right-wing views. In short, cognitive warfare makes heavy use of computational propaganda. Russia and China seized upon the opportunity of the COVID pandemic to increase their operations in cognitive warfare, e.g., to promote various conspiracy theories in the US population to promote the anti-vaxxer campaign.

If left unchecked, pandemics by their very nature lead to security problems (e.g., security breaches at quarantine facilities and overcrowded hospitals, violence at retail outlets due to food shortages, and violent protests against lockdowns). Accordingly, the lack of regulation in cyberspace has not only had the effect of enabling the views of antivaxxers and the like to flourish, thereby undermining vaccination programmes, but it has also caused security problems to arise as a consequence of an uncontrolled pandemic.

It is, of course, impossible to precisely determine the extent to which the COVID-19 virus has been spread knowingly or negligently. However, the number of people, including national leaders, such as former US President Donald Trump and former President of Brazil Jair Bolsonaro, who have through their public stance on vaccination inadvertently facilitated the spread of the virus is presumably in the hundreds of thousands, if not millions. Moreover, pandemics, and certainly COVID-19, create tremendous burdens on critical health infrastructure (e.g., hospitals), cause large-scale economic downturns, and potentially lead to political instability. In short, while pandemics are in the first instance a personal security problem, as well as a safety problem, they are also a potential national security problem.

Governments around the world have used a variety of measures to respond to the COVID-19 pandemic. These measures include identifying the occurrence and spread of an infectious disease in a community – notably, by means of disease reporting requirements, which have traditionally taken place by phone, mail, or fax, but more recently by means of digital disease reporting, including syndromic surveillance (e.g., observance of disease categories identified by means of clusters of symptoms). Other measures seek to stop the spread of the disease by means of economic lockdowns, curfews, border shutdowns, quarantines, contact tracing, social distancing, hand washing, mask wearing, and so on. They also include, crucially, the creation of vaccines to generate a degree of immunity.

An important global institutional framework for combating pandemics is the International Health Regulations (IHRs), which involved the establishment of a global surveillance system for public health emergencies (MacLeish 2017, 70–73). This surveillance system collects and analyses public health data in order to generate information to enable the assessment of threats to public health, notably pandemics, and the determination of appropriate responses to these threats. The system operates locally, nationally and globally. Nation-states are required to notify the WHO of public health emergencies that might transcend national boundaries, e.g., pandemics. According to MacLeish (MacLeish 2017, 71), under the IHRs national sovereignty is subordinated to the derived collective good of global disease surveillance and, ultimately, the collective goods from which it is derived, namely, global public health and global security (and, therefore, national security) in so far as global security relies on global public health. Of course, the IHRs are not enforceable, at least in the case of powerful nations such as China. Nevertheless, the global surveillance system is a clear example of the application of our framework of collective responsibility in the service of a collective good(s).

Cybertechnology, such as metadata and phone apps, has been used for contact tracing. Moreover, there is an important role for big data and associated analytics, including machine-learning techniques, in the prevention and mitigation of pandemics, especially when used in conjunction with whole genome sequencing (WGS) (CDC 2022). This pathogen WGS data can be linked to administrative and other big data, like mobile phone tracking data (GPS) and social media use, to provide very early warning and accurate monitoring during the early stages of disease outbreaks. Moreover, the digitised health and genetic data of populations can be used more generally to identify groups that are particularly vulnerable to specific pathogens, especially when such data is linked with social media data, as well as data about age, location, occupation, and so on. It can also be used for research purposes (e.g., creation of vaccines). However, as we saw in the third section above, there are significant data security risks associated with health and genetic databases and, potentially at least, under certain circumstance these may offset the benefits; certainly these risks need to be mitigated and taken into account.

As also mentioned in the third section above, there is potential utility in sharing health and genetic data stored in databases in the form of a health and medical information commons (HMIC) to combat pandemics. Moreover, our framework of collective goods and associated collective responsibilities is applicable to HMICs. Firstly, there is a collective moral responsibility to combat a pandemic. Secondly, there might be a derived collective moral responsibility to contribute to the creation of such a commons by providing relevant personal data, including not only health and genetic data linked to social media data for research purposes, but also location data from one's smartphone for contact tracing purposes. However, it is important to note that the contribution to the commons should have a defined time horizon and defined connectivity with other data. Thus far, there has not been a great deal of progress in relation to a global health and medical information commons to assist in the control of pandemics. On the other hand, as mentioned above, there have been significant developments in relation to technologically enhanced communicable disease surveillance systems and contact tracing.

Governments have used metadata, apps, social media and messaging services to respond to the COVID-19 pandemic. For instance, South Korea has used phone metadata tracking to directly inform community messaging about the virus (Sorell 2023; Miller and Smith 2023). The government publishes anonymised data of the locations of individuals who have contracted COVID-19, making it available to the public via websites and apps. Text messages are sent to citizens in a specific locality by the health authority. These are very specific and can include anonymised maps of individuals' location history. Depending on the population size of the locality, the specificity of these messages may allow those individuals to be identified, and therefore may infringe upon privacy rights. However, under certain conditions, the collective moral responsibility to combat the pandemic may override individual privacy rights – and, therefore, the right to autonomy, which is constitutive of privacy.

For, as mentioned above, the right to privacy is not absolute; it can be overridden. Moreover, its precise boundaries are unclear. A person does not have a right not to be observed in a public space, but arguably does have a right not to have their movements tracked by their smartphone, even if this right can be overridden under certain circumstances. For instance, this right might be overridden if a person has been directed to self-isolate in a hotel because they have recently returned from overseas – and then only for the purpose of identifying other members of the public who may have been exposed to the virus. Moreover, their right to freedom of movement might also be overridden, given the need for quarantine and, if necessary, enforced quarantine.

What of persons who are carrying the COVID-19 virus and are at a risk of passing it on to other members of the community? Presumably, it is morally acceptable to utilise available data to identify these persons. If so, then it seems morally acceptable to utilise metadata to identify whom these individuals may have contacted, to isolate them, and to provide treatment as early as possible to reduce the chance that they will become ill and possibly die. This will reduce the number of people to whom they will pass the disease.

Evidently, strategies for combating COVID-19 involve a complex set of often competing, and sometimes interconnected (e.g., some privacy rights, such as control over personal data, are themselves aspects of autonomy) moral considerations. Hard choices have to be made. However, the idea of a collective responsibility on the part of individuals to jointly suffer some costs (e.g., loss of privacy rights) in favour of a collective good (e.g., eliminating or containing the spread of COVID-19) lies at the heart of all such effective strategies. This idea provides the theoretical framework for contributing to the collective goods of global public health and security, including, but not restricted to, the prevention and mitigation of pandemics.

Moreover, even if the collection, storage and analysis of health and medical data in an information commons, and the use of metadata or similar tracking and tracing methods, can be morally justified in principle as necessary to avert the threat to the collective good of public health (indeed, global public health) and the collective good of national security (indeed, global security) posed by COVID-19, nevertheless, ethical problems arise from the expanding use of such data for public health surveillance and other security purposes. This is especially the case because of its potential interlinkage with other data available to governments, such as data from social media, biometrics and the rapidly developing capabilities of data analytics and artificial intelligence. First, as already mentioned, and discussed in the third section, these problems include data security risks. Second, the security contexts in which the use of this data is to be permitted might become both very wide and ongoing. For example, the COVID-19 ('biosecurity emergency') context becomes the need to prevent future pandemics and maintain public health more generally; just as, arguably, the 'war' (without end) against terrorism became the war (without end) against serious crime; which, in turn, could at the limit become the 'war' (without end) against crime in general and, in doing so, result in unnecessary and disproportionate curtailment of civil liberties. Third, data, including surveillance data, which was originally and justifiably gathered for one purpose (e.g., taxation or combating a pandemic) is often interlinked with data gathered for another purpose (e.g., crime prevention or in the service of national security), for which there might not be an appropriate justification. Metadata use, in particular, has expanded in some countries, from initially being used by only a few police and security agencies to wide use by governments in many Western countries. This is an example of function creep and illustrates the potential problems that might arise as the threat of COVID-19 eases.

However, as mentioned in the beginning of this section, the public health and national security problems arising from disinformation, computational propaganda and cognitive warfare during a pandemic (and in the overall context of an unregulated cyberspace) might present a moral problem of greater magnitude than either data security risks or potential function creep during and after a pandemic; or at least this might be so for Western liberal democracies.

Dual Use Problems

The history of science and technology is replete with examples of scientific research being used intentionally or unintentionally to create weapons, including WMDs. Scientists have developed chemical, nuclear, cyber and biological weapons. Such weapons include the following historical examples: the mustard gas used by German and British armies in World War 1; the aerial spraying of plague-infested fleas by the Japanese military in World War 2 that killed thousands of Chinese civilians; the dropping of atomic bombs on Hiroshima and Nagasaki by the US Air Force in World War 2; the large-scale biological weapons programme in the Soviet Union from 1946–1992; the biological weapons programme of the apartheid government in South Africa, and; the use of chemical agents against Kurds by Saddam Iraqi Hussein's regime in 1988 and in 2015 by the Assad government in Syria against opposition forces. More recently, cyber-technology has been used to create cyber-weapons which have the potential to cause large-scale harm, e.g. malware used in denial of service attacks. Stuxnet was a worm used to disable Iran's nuclear facilities and, more recently, WannaCry disabled the UK National Health Service's computer systems.

It goes without saying that WMDs are an extraordinary national security threat and, indeed, a global security threat. Therefore, they are, or ought to be, a major focus of NSI agencies. Moreover, of necessity this focus needs not only to be on adversary national security agencies and WMD facilities but on their own relevant facilities and their scientists and engineers. Thus in recent decades there have been a number of high profile 'defections' of scientists from developed liberal demo-cratic states to authoritarian and/or less developed states with WMD programmes. For example, as mentioned above, Abdul Qadeer Khan joined, and in large part established, Pakistan's nuclear weapons programme after working for Urenco in the Netherlands, and Frans van Anraat (also from the Netherlands) went to Iraq to assist Saddam Hussein's WMD programme producing mustard gas.

The security threat posed by WMDs involves various categories of harm and exponentially increases the magnitude of these harms. The 'harms' in question include not only physical and psychological harms to human beings, but also damage to material things, such as artefacts and the physical environment, damage to institutions and, for that matter, to computer software and the like. The security threat posed by WMDs is perhaps most obvious in the case of chemical and nuclear weapons. However, the security threat associated with infectious diseases relating to their potential use in biological weapons is also a major concern. The use of a highly contagious and deadly infectious disease in a biological weapon could lead to an epidemic with catastrophic consequences.

The potential users of WMDs include not only state actors but also non-state actors, such as terrorist groups, nihilistic 'end-of-the-world' groups and, poten-tially, malevolent 'lone-wolf' actors. Of course the threat of the use of some WMDs by some kinds of malevolent actor is far greater than others. The military forces of nation-states with sophisticated R&D programmes are far more likely to use nuclear weapons than non-state actors, at least in the near-term. On the other hand, the use of chemical weapons by non-state actors, such as international terrorist groups, is far more likely than is their use of nuclear weapons. This is in part because of the availability of stockpiles of the relevant toxins and in part because the delivery systems of chemical weapons are relatively unsophisticated. Biological weapons are different again. Much debate regarding the threats posed by biological weapons – and bioterrorism in particular – has focused on the issue of so-called dual-use life science research (NSABB 2015; Miller 2018). While advances in genetics, biotechnology, and synthetic biology may lead to important medical progress, they might also enable production of a new generation of bio-logical weapons of mass destruction. Such dangers are well illustrated by recent research (conducted in the Netherlands and United States) that demonstrated how to produce a strain of avian influenza (H5N1) that is highly contagious among ferrets (which provide the best model for influenza among humans). Due to concerns about the public health and security implications of publishing details about this research, the US National Science Advisory Board for Biosecurity (NSABB), in December 2011, recommended that detailed description of materials and methods be omitted from publications (in science journals) describing the experiments in question (2015). Dual use problems pose a particularly acute problem in relation to national security. On one hand, dual use research ought to be allowed since it is beneficial to humankind. But on the other hand, it is potentially highly dangerous; indeed it can be used to enable WMDs. Let us get greater clarity on the problem of dual use science and technology.

The problem of dual-use ethical dilemmas in relation to powerful, new and emerging technologies, including genomics and biometrics, arises because such technologies have the potential to be used for great harm as well as for great good (Miller and Selgelid, 2007; Miller and Selgelid 2008; van der Bruggen et al. 2011; Tucker 2012; Miller 2013; Miller 2018). As stated above, on the one hand, such technologies can contribute greatly to individual and collective well-being. Consider, for example, nuclear technology that enables the generation of low-cost electricity in populations without obvious alternative energy sources. So nuclear technology is a good thing. On the other hand, these same technologies can be extremely harmful to individuals and collectives; indeed, can be used to create WMDs. Consider, for example, the atomic bombs dropped on Hiroshima and Nagasaki. So it seems that some powerful technologies or, at least, some uses of some powerful technologies, are a bad thing and, therefore, knowledge of these technologies is a bad thing and ignorance a good thing. Accordingly, the question arises as to whether we ought to limit the development of these technologies or, more likely, restrict the uses of these technologies and, in particular, the proliferation of these technologies and perhaps dissemination of the knowledge how to develop them (assuming this is possible).

By definition, dual-use technologies are potentially harmful as well as beneficial, and therefore, there is a need to limit these technologies, or their uses, in a manner that decreases the risk of harm while preserving the benefits. In relation to the potential for harm, governments, regulators, scientists, designers and manufacturers technology and, in the cases of interest to us, law enforcement and national security agencies who use the technology, have a moral responsibility and, specifically a collective or joint moral responsibility, even if not at present a legal responsibility, to cooperate in order to avert or, at least, minimise the risks; so dual use research and technology is a matter of collective moral responsibility to avert or minimise harm. But how does collective responsibility figure in the various scientific, technological and institutional contexts in question? More specifically, should some dual use research and technologies be impermissible or, if not, should certain uses of these technologies be curtailed? More generally, what institutional arrangements, e.g., regulations, ought to be put in place in relation to dual use biometric technologies and uses thereof, specifically in the context of this work by security agencies? We note that given the global threat posed by dual use biometric technology (e.g., virulent transmissible pathogens resulting from gain of function research know no borders) the institutional arrangements require international cooperation; there is a collective moral responsibility on the part to nation states to develop, implement and enforce a global regulatory framework to deal with these dual use problems (and related threats).

'Dual use' refers to scientific research or technology that can be used for both beneficial/good and harmful/bad purposes. However, this general sense of dual use is too broad since it has the effect that almost everything could count as dual use. For instance, machetes are used for farming, but they were also used in the Rwandan genocide in 1994 as tools of murder. So we require a narrower notion of dual use. Most of the current debate has focused on research and technologies with implications not simply for weapons but for weapons of mass destruction (WMDs), in particular – i.e., where the harmful consequences of malevolent use would be on an extremely large scale. That said, defining dual use simply in terms of WMDs yields too narrow a notion given, for instance, the possibility of creating de novo new pathogens which are both highly virulent and highly transmissible (NSABB, 2015; Selgelid, 2016) but might not be weaponised. Accordingly, let us try to get a better fix on a serviceable notion of dual use by setting out a number of different preliminary definitions of dual use familiar in the literature and doing so on the assumption that any definition will involve a degree of stipulation (Miller, 2018 Ch. 1).

Research or technology is dual use if it can be used for:

1 Military and civilian (i.e. non-military) purposes;
2 Beneficial and harmful purposes – where the harmful purposes are to be realised by means of WMDs;
3 Beneficial and harmful purposes – where either the harmful purposes involve the use of weapons as means, and usually WMDs in particular, or the large-scale harm aimed at does not necessarily involve weapons or weaponisation.

In relation to the *purposes* (or ends) of the research, we need to distinguish the following conceptual axes: (i) beneficial/harmful; (ii) military/non-military; and (iii) within the category of military purposes, the sub-categories of offensive/protective. Consider the aerosolisation of a pathogen undertaken for a military purpose. The purpose in question might be offensive, e.g. biowarfare; but it might simply be protective, e.g. to understand the nature and dangers of such aerosolisation in order to prepare protections against an enemy known to be planning to deploy the aerosolised pathogen in question as a weapon.

The categories beneficial/harmful and military/non-military do not necessarily mirror one another. Some non-military purposes are, nevertheless, harmful, e.g. the supplier of a vaccine releasing a pathogen to make large numbers of people sick in order that the sick buy the vaccine against the pathogen and, thereby, increase the supplier's profits. And some military purposes might be good, e.g. the above-mentioned research on the aerosolisation of a pathogen undertaken for purely protective purposes in the context of a morally justified war. The United States Project BioShield is an example of research aimed at providing 'new tools to improve medical countermeasures protecting Americans against a chemical, biological, radiological or nuclear (CBRN) attack' (USDHSS 2004). However, some of the protective research would probably yield results that could assist in the development and delivery of biological weapons.

Notice that in the case of GOF research, such as research that enables the creation of a highly virulent pathogen that is transmissible to humans, the researchers (presumably) do not have a malevolent purpose (Selgelid 2016). Perhaps they want to understand the process by means of which such a virulent pathogen might mutate and put humans at risk having as an ultimate end to create a vaccine against such a transmissible pathogen. Nevertheless, these researchers have in fact created a highly dangerous new pathogen which has the potential to be intentionally released into a human population by persons other than the researchers. Accordingly, such GOF research is dual use on our definition, notwithstanding that it does not involve an explicit process of weaponisation.

In light of the discussion thus far, it is clear that there is a need for the implementation of a significant array of regulatory measures in the biological sciences in respect of dual use issues, albeit not over-regulation to the point that, so to speak, the baby is thrown out with the bathwater. Moreover, those with responsibilities in this regard are many. They include not only researchers, but institutional managers, members of governments and, for that matter, citizens. Accordingly, and given what is at stake, there is a collective moral responsibility in this regard. These measures ought to be integrated such that taken together they constitute a web of prevention; so the collective moral responsibility is to be institutionally embedded in a web of prevention comprised of various regulatory measures. Such measures include the imposition of limits on dual-use experiments and on the dissemination of potentially dangerous information resulting from dual-use discoveries. Moreover, the national security threat posed by dual use research in the biological sciences, NSI agencies need to have a critical role in relation to the development and implementation of these regulatory measures and, of course, in ensuring that the regulations are being complied with both nationally and, in so far as it is possible, internationally.

Some obvious regulatory measures that should be considered include the following ones identified by Miller (Miller 2018: 112–113) and Miller and Selgelid (2007) (see also van der Bruggen, Miller and Selgelid 2011): regulations providing for mandatory physical safety and security of the storage, transport and physical access to samples of pathogens, equipment, laboratories etc.; licensing of a limited number of laboratories to engage in research involving dual-use technologies; vetting of researchers; censorship constraints, e.g., research findings might need to be disseminated in such a way that anyone being informed of these findings would not be able to replicate the experiments that enabled the results reported in the findings; an international agreement on safety and security procedures in the biological sciences, including but not restricted to dual use issues and export controls worldwide; verification procedures should be added to the Biological and Toxin Weapons Convention.

As noted above, there is a collective moral responsibility on the part of nation states to implement and enforce a set of regulations, such as the ones just proposed. However, there is a collective action problem with respect to a number of these, including the requirement for verification procedures. Nation-states are adversaries in the development of technology and, in some instances, adversaries to the point of waging war, as the Russian invasion of Ukraine and NATO's support of Ukraine, demonstrates. Moreover, as noted above, there is a history of biological warfare programmes. In this adversarial international context, international cooperation confronts a collective action problem (Miller 2013). On the one hand, it is in the collective interest to cooperate in relation to dual use problems in the biological sciences to prevent massive collective harm in the form of, for instance, a catastrophic pandemic or biowarfare and the proliferation of biological weapons. On the other hand, it might be in the interest of each, or at least some, to free-ride, i.e., to press ahead with dangerous dual use research or to develop a 'defensive' biowarfare programme.

Conclusion

The focus of this chapter has been on biosecurity problems that constitute national security problems and, therefore, require national security intelligence activity and, specifically, the ethical dimension of such national security intelligence activity. We have provided conceptual distinctions between biosecurity and biosafety, and between national security and national interest, and introduced a normative framework based on the concepts of collective moral goods and collective moral responsibility. We have discussed in general terms three fundamental problems with an ethical dimension, namely data security (broadly construed), pandemic control and dual use issues. Each of these issues deserves much greater attention than could be given in a single book chapter. Moreover, we have not addressed a number of important biosecurity problems with an ethical dimension. For instance. we have not addressed directly and in detail bioterrorism and biowarfare, although each of the three problems that are discussed have important implications for combating bioterrorism and biowarfare. In relation to dual use problems in the biological sciences, we have focused on developments in synthetic biology in respect of pathogens. However, the so-called CRISPR revolution involves gene editing in respect of humans and, as such, brings with it an array of acute ethical problems. The analysis of these will need to be left for another day.

References

Albright, David and Hinderstein, Corey. 2004. "Unravelling the A Q Khan and Future Proliferation Networks". Washington *Quarterly.* 28: 1. /www.twq.com/05spring/index.cfm?id=147. Accessed: 23/4/2024.

Cassels, Jamie. 1991. "The Uncertain Promise of Law: Lessons from Bhopal". *Osgoode Hall Law Journal.* 29: 1, 1–50.

Cassidy, Caitlin. 2024. "Alice Springs Youth Curfew". *Guardian Newspaper*, 27 March. www.theguardian.com/australia-news/2024/mar/27/alice-springs-brawl-teenager-death-todd-tavern. Accessed: 20/4/2024.

Centre for Counterproliferation Research (CCR). 2002. *Anthrax in America: A Chronology and Analysis of the 2001 Attacks.* Washington, DC: National Defense University. https://wmdcenter.ndu.edu/Portals/97/Documents/Publications/Articles/Anthrax-in-America.pdf

Centers for Disease Control and Prevention (CDC). 2022. "What is Whole Genome Sequencing (WGS)". www.cdc.gov/pulsenet/pathogens/wgs.htm. Accessed: 28/4/2024.

Collier, Roger. 2017. "NHS Ransomware Attack Spreads Worldwide". *CMAJ.* 189: 22. www.ncbi.nlm.nih.gov/pmc/articles/PMC5461132/. Accessed: 23/4/2024.

Coto, Danica. 2024. "Haitian Capital Seeks to Revive Its Heyday as Gang Violence Consumes Port-au-Prince". *Associated Press*, 20 April 2024. https://apnews.com/article/haiti-cap-haitien-capital-gangs-violence-3e101149ced94ce0da41d9621234f41c. Accessed: 28/4/2024.

Davis, Jessica. 2021. "Surveillance, Intelligence and Ethics in a COVID-19 World". In Miller, S., Regan, M., and Walsh, P. F. (eds.) 2021. *NSI and Ethics*. London: Routledge. 156–165.

Feltes, Jonas. 2021. "Collective Responsibility and Chemical, Biological, Radiological and Nuclear Terrorism". In Miller, S., Feltes, J., and Henschke, A. (eds.). *Counter-Terrorism: The Ethical Issues*. Cheltenham, UK: Edward Elgar. 181–194.

Henschke, Adam, Miller, Seumas, Walsh, Patrick F., and Bradbury, Roger. 2024. *The Ethics of NSI Institutions: Theory and Practice*. London: Routledge.

Macnish, Kevin and Henschke, Adam (eds.) 2023. *The Ethics of Surveillance in Times of Emergency*. Oxford: Oxford University Press.

McLeish, Caitriona. 2017. "Evolving Biosecurity Frameworks". In Dover, R., Dylan, H., and Goodman, M. (eds.). *The Palgrave Handbook of Security, Risk and Intelligence*. London: Palgrave-Macmillan. 63–78.

Miller, Seumas. 2001. *Social Action: A Teleological Account*. New York: Cambridge University Press.

Miller, Seumas. 2009. *Terrorism and Counter-terrorism: Ethics and Liberal Democracy*. Oxford: Blackwell Publishing.

Miller, Seumas. 2010. *The Moral Foundations of Social Institutions: A Philosophical Study*. New York: Cambridge University Press.

Miller, Seumas. 2013. "Moral Responsibility, Collective Action Problems and the Dual Use Dilemma in Science and Technology". In Rappert, B. and Selgelid, M. (eds.). *On the Dual Uses of Science and Ethics: Principles, Practices and Prospects*. Canberra: ANU Press. 185–206.

Miller, Seumas. 2018. *Dual Use Science and Technology, Ethics and Weapons of Mass Destruction*. Dordrecht: Springer.

Miller, Seumas. 2021. "Rethinking the Just Intelligence Theory of NSI Collection and Analysis: Principles of Discrimination, Necessity, Proportionality and Reciprocity". *Social Epistemology.* 35: 3, 211–231.

Miller, Seumas. 2022. "NSI Activity: A Philosophical Analysis". *Intelligence and National Security.* 37: 6, 791–808.

Miller, Seumas. 2023. "Cognitive Warfare: An Ethical Analysis". *Ethics and Information Technology.* 25: 3. https://doi.org/10.1007/s10676-023-09717-7. Accessed: 28/4/2024.

Miller, Seumas and Bossomaier, Terry. 2024. *Cybersecurity, Ethics and Collective Responsibility*. New York: Oxford University Press.

Miller, Seumas and Feltes, Jonas. 2021. "Collective Responsibility and Counter-Terrorism". In Miller, S., Feltes, J., and Henschke, A. (eds.). *Counter-Terrorism: The Ethical Issues*. Cheltenham, UK: Edward Elgar. 35–45.

Miller, Seumas and Selgelid, Michael. 2007. "Ethical and Philosophical Consideration of the Dual Use Dilemma in the Biological Sciences". *Science and Engineering Ethics.* 13: 523–580.

Miller, Seumas and Selgelid, Michael. 2008. *Ethical and Philosophical Consideration of the Dual Use Dilemma in the Biological Sciences*. Dordrecht: Springer.

Miller, Seumas and Smith, Marcus. 2021. "Ethics, Public Health and Technology Responses to COVID-19". *Bioethics.* 35: 4, 366–371.

Miller, Seumas and Smith, Marcus. 2022. "Quasi-Universal Forensic DNA Databases". *Criminal Justice Ethics.* 41: 3, 238–256.

Miller, Seumas and Smith, Marcus. 2023. "Combating COVID 19: Surveillance, Autonomy and Collective Responsibility". In Macnish, K. and Henschke, A. (eds.), *The Ethics of Surveillance in Times of Emergency*. Oxford: Oxford University Press. 47–59.

Mueller, Robert. 2019. *Report in the Investigation into Russian Interference in the 2016 US Presidential Election*. Washington, DC: US Department of Justice.

National Human Genome Research Institute (NHGRI). 2019. *A Brief Guide to Genomics*. www.genome.gov/about-genomics/fact-sheets/A-Brief-Guide-to-Genomics. Accessed: 20/4/2024.

National Science Advisory Board for Biosecurity (NSABB). 2015. *Framework for Conducting Risk and Benefit Assessments of Gain-of-Function Research*. Washington, DC: NSABB.

Qiang, Xiao. 2019. "The Road to Digital Unfreedom: President Xi's Surveillance State". *Journal of Democracy.* 30: 1, 53–67.

Rabinowitz, Hannah. 2023. "FBI Director Wray Acknowledges Bureau Assessment that COVID-19 Likely Resulted from Lab Incident". *CNN,* 1 March. https://edition.cnn.com/2023/02/28/politics/wray-fbi-covid-origins-lab-china/index.html. Accessed: 23/4/2024.

Rioss, Elias. 2022. "DNA Dystopia". *Brooklyn Law Review*. 87: 4.

Selgelid, Michael. 2016. "Gain of Function Research: Ethical Analysis". *Science and Engineering Ethics.* 22: 4, 923–964.

Shoham, Dany and Wolfson, Ze'ev. 2004. "The Russian Biological Weapons Program". *Critical Reviews in Microbiology*. 30: 4, 241–261.

Smith, Marcus. 2018. "Universal Forensic DNA Databases: Balancing the Costs and Benefits". *Alternative Law Journal.* 43: 2, 131–135.

Smith, Marcus and Miller, Seumas. 2021. *Biometric Identification, Law and Ethics*. Dordrecht: Springer.

Sorell, Tom. 2023. "Pandemic Population Surveillance: Privacy and Life-Saving". In Macnish, K. and Henschke, A. (eds.). *Surveillance in Times of Emergency*. Oxford: Oxford University Press. 15–29.

Tucker, Jonathan (ed.). 2012. *Innovation, Dual Use and Security: Managing the Risk of Emerging Biological and Chemical Technologies*. Harvard, MA: MIT Press.

US Department of Health and Human Services (USDHHS). 2004. "HHS Fact Sheet Project Bioshield". *DHHS,* 21 July 2004. (www.hhs.gov/news/press/2004pres/20040721b.html. Accessed: 28/4/2024.

Van der Bruggen, Koos, Miller, Seumas, and Selgelid, Michael. 2011. *Report on Biosecurity and Dual Use Research*. The Hague: Dutch Research Council.

Walsh, Patrick F. 2018. *Intelligence, Biosecurity and Bioterrorism*. London: Palgrave-Macmillan.

Walsh, Patrick F. 2021. "Evolving Chemical, Biological, Radiological and Nuclear (CBRN) Terrorism: Intelligence Community Response and Ethical Challenges". In Miller, S., Regan, M., and Walsh, P. F. (eds.). *NSI and Ethics*. London: Routledge. 261–279.

Walsh, Patrick F., James Ramsay, and Ausma Bernot. 2023. "Health Security Intelligence Capabilities Post COVID-19: Resisting the Passive 'New Normal' within the Five Eyes". *Intelligence and National Security.* 38: 7, 1095–1111.

Walsh, Patrick F and Miller, Seumas. 2016. "Rethinking 'Five-Eyes' Security Intelligence Collection Policies and Practices Post 9/11/Post-Snowden". *Intelligence and National Security*. 31: 3, 345–368.

Woods, M. and Pringle, J. 2022. "Ontario Premier Says, 'Ottawa Under Siege' and Declares State of Emergency". *CTV News*. https://ottawa.ctvnews.ca/freedom-convoy-2022. Accessed: 30/10/23.

8 Improving the Health Security Intelligence Workforce and Research Agenda

Kathleen M. Vogel

Introduction

The COVID-19 pandemic has illustrated the current and future need for incorporating health security intelligence knowledge and expertise into the intelligence community (IC) workforce. Traditionally, expertise in health security has not been a driver in the hiring and professional development of intelligence practitioners. In general, this state of affairs is because Patrick Walsh writes, "historically ICs have not had a good understanding of bio-threats and risks from the Cold War up to and after the Coalition invasion of Iraq in 2003" (Walsh 2020, 586). To better understand natural, accidental, and deliberate causes of disease outbreak and transmission, health security expertise, ranges from the biological and life sciences, medicine, public health, animal health, epidemiology, physical sciences, data/information science, public policy, humanities, and the social sciences (Morens et al. 2020; Wilson & McNamara, 2020; Jehn et al., 2022; Seth 2018; Desclaux & Anoko 2017; Smith et al. 2019; Taylor 2019; Bernard et al. 2021; Ross et al. 2021; Bernard & Sullivan 2020).

It can also encompass specialized expertise related to biological weapons (e.g., how different state and non-state actors have developed and used biological weapons), as well as the intersection between disease and war/conflicts, and how these issues could pose additional types of health security threats (Wheelis 2000; Smallman-Raynor & Cliff 2004; Geissler & van Courtland Moon 1999; Guillemin 1999). There has been recognition that currently the number of worldwide bioweapons experts, who have deep knowledge of former weapons programs, is diminishing due to aging/retirement, death, and a lack of career opportunities for young professionals. All of this, coupled with the fact that more new emerging diseases are expected to appear worldwide due to climate change, displaced populations, conflict, a rise in antimicrobial drug resistance, globalization, and other factors, we can expect the demand for health security intelligence to rise—particularly within intelligence communities as they are tasked with identifying security threats to the homeland (Office of the Director of National Intelligence 2023; National Intelligence Council 2021). The key question then becomes how to start inculcating and building up health security expertise within intelligence communities now and in the years to come. It should be stated, however, that although

DOI: 10.4324/9781003335511-11

greater engagement with, and development of, health security expertise by the IC is desirable, it remains to be seen whether national governments and their intelligence agencies might prioritize such initiatives. In spite of this, it is useful to consider different approaches that one could take to guide IC workforce development strategy for health security—each has pros and cons that would need to be considered by intelligence officials. These will be outlined in the sections below.

Building Health Security Expertise and Knowledge within Intelligence Communities

To date, there have been a series of debates within intelligence communities about whether intelligence practitioners should be "generalists" (have broad knowledge, be able to work on many different accounts, and able to be fungible) or "specialists" (able to have particular expertise that they apply to a specific work account for extended periods of time). Historically, specialists, particularly within the analytic cadre, have dominated intelligence community practices. This was true, for example, in the United States through much of the Cold War. However, starting in the 1970s and more acutely after the Cold War ended and the rise of concerns over new state and non-state actor threats in the 1990s, U.S. IC management preferred to train and hire analysts who were generalists so that they could be adaptable for whatever security threat might arise (Russell 2007). This preference has intensified in subsequent decades, such that now the generalist model for hiring and promotion is dominant in the U.S. intelligence analytic cadre. Although the generalist model can allow for more management flexibility, it can also be a contributing factor to producing erroneous threat assessments when important expertise is not available or used, as was seen in the intelligence failures leading up to the 2003 Iraq war (Vogel 2013; Kerr et al. 2005).

Discussions about future intelligence workforce needs on health security demand that IC officials consider the implications of whether a "generalist" or "specialist" hiring strategy is pursued. As noted above, the multi-disciplinary nature of health security intelligence means that regardless of which intelligence community (IC) workforce strategy, or combinations of strategy, are chosen, there will be a need to incorporate a range of disciplinary knowledge and expertise as health security threats arise (Lentzos et al. 2020).

If one adopts a specialist model, a first approach could be to launch a hiring priority on health security expertise to augment the existing IC analytic workforce. These hires could be positioned within different regional or functional units within IC analysis and collection. An alternative approach would be to create new centers within the IC where this specialized expertise is housed, similar to how the U.S. Central Intelligence Agency (CIA) has recently created a new Directorate of Digital Innovation and a new China Mission Center to focus attention and expertise on these high priority issues (Central Intelligence Agency n.d.a; Marquardt 2021). Interestingly, in December 2022, the U.S. Department of State announced that it would establish the Bureau of Global Health Security and Diplomacy to strengthen its capabilities in preparing and responding to global health security threats

(Blinken 2022). One can anticipate that the State Department's intelligence arm, the Bureau of Intelligence and Research, would also play some role in this new Bureau although this remains to be revealed.

More opportunities for professional development among the IC workforce could be created to support either generalists or specialists that would involve academic outreach. IC analysts could spend rotations at universities to learn about different knowledge sets and analytic techniques related to projecting future health security threats or deepen their existing knowledge about health security issues from institutions such as the WHO Collaborating Center for Global Health Security at Johns Hopkins University (Arizona State University, n.d.; World Health Organization, n.d.). There is also the IC's Public-Private Talent Exchange (PPTE) program, which provides IC personnel opportunities to engage with private sector partners and learn new skills and expertise (Office of the Director of National Intelligence, n.d.); these could be applied to private sector entities with expertise in health security collection and analysis (e.g., pharmaceutical or biotechnology industries, biosurveillance and data analytics companies). To support these rotations/details, there need to be new promotion and reward opportunities for IC practitioners, and also a more flexible work routine to allow it. The COVID-19 pandemic has opened the door for more flexible work arrangements, including remote work and there are various IC debates about if these would continue in the future (Danoy 2021; Landon-Murray & Anderson 2021; Gioe et al. 2020). These arrangements, however, would provide analysts with more opportunities and flexibility to meet and talk to experts on the outside and attend relevant health security meetings, seminars and other educational opportunities to build their health security expertise in-house. However, it should be recognized that not all health security needs should be built within the IC—the ICs of any country could work to collaborate more with public health agencies and other public health experts to augment its in-house capabilities (e.g., reaching out to national academies of science members for specific technical questions). In turn, external outreach by the IC to public health experts could enhance the ability of the public health community to better understand national security concerns, as well as national security approaches to threat assessment, such as early warning methods.

Another parallel approach would be to draw on relevant outside experts and bring them into the IC for short- or long-term postings. The State Department's Bureau of Intelligence and Research's Analytic Exchange program convenes leading experts from academia, thinktanks, nongovernmental organizations (NGOs), and private industry worldwide to participate in meetings, workshops, seminars on IC-relevant topics (U.S. Department of State Bureau of Intelligence and Research, n.d.). There is also the Jefferson Science Fellowship program (run by the U.S. National Academies of Science) that brings in tenured professors from American universities into the U.S. Department of State to work for one-year in a variety of bureaus, including the Bureau of Intelligence and Research (INR), one of seventeen intelligence agencies within the U.S. IC (U.S. National Academies of Science, Engineering, and Medicine n.d.). Moreover, the CIA has also launched a new CIA Technology Fellows program to bring promising experts to the agency for one to two years of public service (Harris 2021).

In contrast to the United States, Patrick Walsh has noted, the Australian Intelligence Community, "has been more insular and risk adverse in its approach to external research collaboration than other Five Eyes partners such as the US and Canada" (Walsh 2016, 14). In 2018, the Office of National Intelligence in Australia created an emergent academic outreach program, but it is still under development and a more formalized program is needed. While some progress in the last couple of years is evident, it is unclear whether health security will be considered within this program (Walsh 2022). Australia also has a national intelligence science advisory board, which includes senior IC managers, and prominent STEM and social science academics for advising on where research priorities should be invested (Walsh 2022); this advisory board could consider research priorities in the health security space. In Canada, the Canadian Security Intelligence Service (CSIS) has had for many years its Academic Outreach and Stakeholder Engagement program, which has periodically engaged with the academic and research community through various workshops and meetings; although these programs have not focused on biological threats or health security, more opportunities here could be geared potentially towards relevant health security issues (Government of Canada 2022; Tiernan 2017, 147–62).

On the research front, there are also opportunities for outside experts to work on health-security related intelligence projects relevant to the U.S. IC, such as in the CIA Labs which was created in 2020 to bring together CIA officers together with the private sector and academics to conduct research on science and technology matters that relate to CIA interests (Central Intelligence Agency, n.d.b), as well as the Intelligence Advanced Research Projects Agency (IARPA). For example, IARPA has sponsored a series of research programs around COVID-19 (Intelligence Advanced Research Projects Agency, n.d.). Also, the IC Associates program enables academics to work with the IC on a contractual basis and conduct studies/white papers/consultations related to IC topics of interest (The Intelligence Community Inc, n.d.).

Moreover, there are existing national research collaboration programs available among the "Five Eyes" (Australia, Canada, New Zealand, the United Kingdom and the United States) that could promote more work on health security intelligence: These include the U.S./UK NSF-UKRI partnership to promote collaborations between U.S. and U.K. academic scholars; these projects could involve topics related to health security issues involving both technical and social science expertise (National Science Foundation, 2022; UK Research and Innovation, 2022). There is also an NSF–Canada research partnership that could be expanded to include health security topics of mutual interest (National Science Foundation, 2021). In Australia, its Office of National Intelligence (ONI) set up about two years ago a National Intelligence and Security Discovery Research Grants (Intelligence Challenges) scheme, which is administered currently by the Australian Research Council, but funded via the ONI, which could support health security "challenges." Indeed, in a recent funding round, ONI identified "emerging biological and materials science exploitation challenges" as one of its key research priorities, which funding research that can improve the ability of Australia's IC to "detect, identify, analyse, counter, defeat and prosecute threats" from emerging biotechnologies (Office of National Intelligence 2023). The Australian Department of Defence National Security Science and Technology Centre (NSSTC) has a similar scheme to support research of national security and intelligence interest. A national social science intelligence research group, with various interest sub-groups focused on social and behavioral sciences has also been established in Australia, but it is still in preliminary stages (Walsh 2022). In addition, there was a recent Australian CSIRO-U.S. NSF research collaboration program on artificial intelligence (CSIRO, 2022); a similar type of funding call could be developed for health security issues. There could also be other relevant agencies across the "Five Eyes" that could fund research in health security intelligence. For example, the U.S. Office of Naval Research Global with the U.S. Embassy in Singapore sponsors research collaborations between U.S. and Singaporean scientists (Office of Naval Research n.d.; U.S. Embassy Singapore 2021); one could imagine health security issues relevant to the Asia region being supported through this type of program.

Beyond IC–academia interactions, there are also useful roles that the larger area of Open Source Intelligence (OSINT) can play. The IC defines open source information (either in verbal, written, or electronic form) as that which can be obtained legally, for instance from the Internet, a human source, or physical locations that US or allied forces have taken control over (Richelson 2015). Open source information can include, in electronic or non-electronic form, various categories, such as: (1) traditional media (e.g., foreign and domestic television, radio, and print media); (2) information obtained via the Internet which includes online publications, online reviews, blogs, discussion groups, citizen media and user generated content (e.g., people taking pictures with their cell phones and posting them), YouTube, and social media and networking sites (e.g., Facebook, LinkedIn, Instagram, Twitter), online discussion groups such as Reddit, bookmarking sites such as Pinterest, and E-Commerce such as Amazon; (3) public government data (e.g., government reports, budgets, hearings, telephone directories, press conferences, websites, speeches); (4) professional/industry/academic publications and commercial data (e.g., commercial imagery, financial and industrial assessments, databases); (5) seized foreign material; (6) grey literature, including foreign or domestic open source material that is usually only available through specialized channels and may not enter normal channels or systems of publication, distribution, bibliographic control, or acquisition by booksellers or subscription agents (e.g., technical reports, patents, business documents) (Richelson 2015; Henricks 2017).

Although greater OSINT capabilities on health security issues could be cultivated within the IC, there are also many private sector actors who could be hired to contractually provide this expertise and capacity to the IC. For example, there are OSINT entities such as Bellingcat, which is a Dutch-based investigative journalism group using a variety of online sources, as well as data science techniques to investigate security-related issues. Bellingcat has conducted open source research to dispel a variety of disinformation campaigns and cyber-attacks related to the COVID-19 pandemic (Koryakina & Jolokhava 2020; Tian 2020; Antonova 2020). Entities such as Bellingcat could also help the IC assess and refute various Russian disinformation campaigns about U.S. origins of disease outbreaks and bioweapons activities (Lentzos & Littlewood 2022). Finally, there are other private sector companies that collect open source information about local disease outbreaks worldwide in order to anticipate surges indicating an epidemic or pandemic (Wilson 2016; Wilson 2018; Wilson et al. 2022).

Regardless of which strategy/approach is pursued, a recent RAND study notes that there are important considerations for IC workforce planning that can serve as guideposts for the future: (1) rebuilding lost (or largely absent in the health security case) capability takes time, (2) resource flexibility is needed, (3) risk is an essential element in workforce planning, (4) systematic planning shores up requirements (Nemfakos 2013). Intelligence communities should start strategizing now about how they will build up health security workforce needs. It is clear that with many current and future environmental and geopolitical changes that health security threats will be with us for the long-haul and it is in the IC's interests to start planning for new outreach, workforce additions, and professional development to address these threats on the horizon.

Organizational Questions and Potential Challenges

As noted above, there exist a variety of opportunities and mechanisms for either building in health security intelligence expertise within the IC or creating new conduits for acquiring this expertise from the outside. New initiatives could be launched, with new funding to support this agenda. However, there are potential intelligence organizational issues that would need to be resolved to ensure the effectiveness of these new initiatives. Organizationally, who/what should be the focal point for health security intelligence? How should it be organized internally compared to other important mission areas? Typically, one way to focus attention and resources on new threats in the IC is to create "Centers." However, one downside is that these approaches may not inculcate health security expertise more broadly across different regional and functional bureaus/units. Or, alternatively, one could consider creating smaller, innovative units within different parts of the IC as has been done for other emerging/ experimental issues (Vogel and Tyler, 2019). These kinds of units, however, tend to be fragile, and require a variety of high level leadership and organizational supports to last long term.

This gets to the larger issue of who would "own" or have authority over health security intelligence within the IC or should health security intelligence be seen as a cross-cutting issue? More often than not, health security intelligence would likely be housed within units that work on biological weapons issues—but is that the right home in intelligence moving forward? Health security intelligence encompasses issues that go beyond purely deliberate attacks. Also, in many cases, it can be difficult to know the attribution of an unusual disease outbreak in the early stages, and so all possible origins need to be investigated. Thus, in a more provocative move, it is useful to consider: should health security intelligence be the main organizing umbrella for all biological threats within intelligence? Under this formulation, biological weapons threats or other kinds of deliberate attacks involving biological materials would only be one of several threats considered for intelligence involving biological issues. This umbrella health security arrangement would allow for episodes like disease outbreaks and epidemics around the world to receive more intelligence attention and resources than they have had in the past. Resolving this issue of who owns health security intelligence might also help to ward off turf issues or help to resolve conflicts when difference of opinion/dissent arise among different intelligence experts about the nature of a health security threat. This problem was seen with the U.S. intelligence community's assessment of the COVID-19 origins, in which the IC was divided between two camps: those who believed the data on the virus were consistent with a laboratory-associated incident and those who believed the data were more consistent with a natural exposure to an infected animal (Office of the Director of National Intelligence/National Intelligence Council 2021; Pollard and Kuznar 2022, 17–24).

As diseases do not respect borders, there is also a need to develop greater coordination, collaboration, and information sharing mechanisms across the Five Eyes on health security intelligence. This could take a variety of forms. For example, the "Five Eyes" could organize regular health security intelligence exercises (e.g., audit/after action reports, forecasting/backcasting exercises, scenario planning) to promote learning and analytic best practices. The "Five Eyes" already organize regular annual/semi-annual meetings among bioweapons experts; one could think about using a similar model or mechanism to organize regular health security meetings among the "Five Eyes" that would also involve a broader array of health security experts. In the next section I will discuss what a health security research agenda could look like within and across the Five Eyes.

An Emergent Health Security Research Agenda

I will end this chapter by focusing attention on six key areas that would benefit from prioritized research by the IC in the health security domain. Any agenda of course is dependent on whether "Five Eyes" ICs see the need for resourcing or supporting these research areas as their attention inevitably begins to shift to managing other threats and risks post COVID-19. Actual engagement with health security issues by each "Five Eyes" ICs will depend on the culture and mission of their ICs, and political expectations, including the framing of intelligence priorities. Nonetheless, IC capability can be built by investing in: (1) effects of climate change; (2) emerging bio-science/technology; (3) bio-data/algorithmic security risks; (4) dis/misinformation; (5) resolving health security disputes among experts; and (6) early warning systems. First, it is clear that the varying effects of climate change (changing temperatures and precipitation patterns) have caused the increase of a variety of pathogens worldwide, including into new geographic areas that pose risks to human and animal health. We need better understandings at both the micro- and macro-levels of combined scientific and social science data that reveal more specifically how climate change is affecting particular populations of pathogens and their interactions with human and animal hosts. Second, with advances in life science research, there are continually new scientific and technological breakthroughs (e.g., genome editing, creation of potential pandemic pathogens) that can pose increased risks to human and animal health through either accidental or intentional release of pathogens from a laboratory. In this domain, we also need more clear understandings of how the skills associated with these advances are democratizing and becoming available to a wider community of potential users, and also how, in some cases, what scientific skills are still difficult to master or replicate. This research will help security agencies better determine what scientific and technological developments are worth the time, effort, and resources to worry about.

Third, with the increased use of big data and algorithms in biological science work, there are growing concerns about the current and future risks of malicious exploitation at the interface of advanced data analytics and artificial intelligence/ machine learning technologies with genomic and other kinds of biological data. With the increasing digitalization of biology, we need more research on the health security risks that can stem from the use of bio-data. Fourth, related to bio-data in its various forms, it is clear from the COVID-19 pandemic and public debates about vaccination, that there are a number of state and non-state actors who choose to use (whether knowingly or unintentionally) misinformation or disinformation to spread falsehoods about health security issues (Bernard et al. 2021; Ling 2022; Winter et al. 2021). A new research agenda in this space would focus on how to detect and counter health mis/disinformation campaigns. Fifth, the COVID-19 pandemic has further shown the challenges of how to resolve disputes among experts working in various health security domains. Scientific, public health, and intelligence communities have struggled to research and analyze the origins of the COVID-19 pandemic to determine whether it was a natural outbreak or one stemming from accidental release from a laboratory. Future pathogen outbreaks that arise may also face these same challenges to identify the origins of the outbreak. More technical and social science research is needed to better sort through disparate pieces of data and claims, as well as how to reconcile opposing views on health security threats when the data remains inconclusive or contradictory. Finally, for whatever pathogens might arise in the future, we need better indicators and early warning detection systems using classified and unclassified information to be able to identify more quickly and accurately potential health security threats as they arise. From a health security perspective, each of these six areas are expected to remain priority concerns in the years and decades to come so it will be money well spent for governments to invest and build up research capabilities in these areas in anticipation of, and to better counter, the next set of health security threats.

Conclusion

Shortly after 9/11, biosecurity scholar Gerald Epstein (2001) wrote, "The biological research community, the biotech industry, and the national security community do not share a history of interaction that has characterized other disciplines such as microelectronics, computer science, or space technology" (pp. 321–322). Even more nascent is the public health sector–IC relationship—which has typically been more sporadic/ad-hoc and usually focused on disease threats of soldiers/ forces deployed abroad (Bowsher et al. 2016; Baker et al. 2020). Health security expertise related to intelligence matters has also been brought to bear on specific types of deliberate bioweapons incidents, such as the Sverdlovsk anthrax outbreak (Guillemin 1999), the yellow rain controversy (Guillemin et al. 1985), smallpox threat assessments in the 1990s (Henderson et al. 1999), bioterrorism incidents (Torok et al. 1997), or more recently, gain-of-function experiments (Tilley 2022). These past examples have tended to be ad-hoc and more reactionary outreach efforts when a controversy arises—what is needed is a more long-term workforce strategy that would allow for more timely expertise to be brought to bear on the next health security intelligence problem. As Sue Gordon, the former Principal Deputy Director of the Director of National Intelligence states, "When the nature of the national security threat changes, intelligence must change" (Dilanian 2020). Now is the time to start building health security capacity within intelligence.

References

Antonova, N. (2020). *"Satanic" Vaccines and Satire Gone Wild: COVID-19 Disinfo Meets Religion.* Retrieved from www.bellingcat.com/news/2020/04/15/satanic-vaccines-and-satire-gone-wild-covid-19-disinfo-meets-religion/

Arizona State University (n.d.). *Threatcasting Lab.* Retrieved from https://threatcasting.asu.edu/

Baker, M.S., Kevany, S., Canyon, D., & Baker, J. (2020). The intersection of global health, military medical intelligence, and national security in the management of transboundary hazards and outbreaks. *Security Nexus*, 1–9. Retrieved from www.jstor.org/stable/resrep25704?seq=1#metadata_info_tab_contents

Bernard, E., Bowsher, G., Sullivan, R., & Gibson-Fall, F. (2021). Disinformation and epidemics: Anticipating the next phase of biowarfare. *Health Security*, *19*(1), 3–12. http://doi.org/10.1089/hs.2020.0038

Bernard, R. & Sullivan, R. (2020). The use of HUMINT in epidemics: A practical assessment. *Intelligence and National Security*, *35*(4), 493–501. http://doi.org/10.1080/02684527.2020.1750137

Blinken, A.J. (2022). *Plans for a Bureau of Global Health Security and Diplomacy.* Retrieved from www.state.gov/plans-for-a-bureau-of-global-health-security-and-diplomacy/

Bowsher, G., Milner, C., & Sullivan, R. (2016). Medical intelligence, security, and global health: The foundations of a new health agenda. *Journal of the Royal Society of Medicine*, *109*(7), 269–273. http://doi.org/10.1177/0141076816656483

Central Intelligence Agency (n.d.a). *Directorate of Digital Innovation.* Retrieved from www.cia.gov/about/organization/#directorate-of-digital-innovation

Central Intelligence Agency (n.d.b). *CIA Labs*. Retrieved from www.cia.gov/cia-labs/

CSIRO (2022). *CSIRO-National Science Foundation (US) AI Research Collaboration Program*. Retrieved from www.csiro.au/en/research/technology-space/ai/NSF-AI-Research

Danoy, J. (2021). The U.S. Intelligence Community's Complicated Relationship with Telework. *The Cipher Brief*. Retrieved from www.thecipherbrief.com/the-us-intellige nce-communitys-complicated-relationship-with-telework

Desclaux, A. & Anoko, J. (2017). L'anthropologie engagée dans la lutte contre Ebola (2014–2016): Approches, contributions et nouvelles questions [Anthropology engaged against Ebola (2014–2016): Approches, contributions and new questions]. *Sante Publique*, *29*(4), 477–485. http://doi.org/10.3917/spub.174.0477

Dilanian, K. (2020). Coronavirus may force the U.S. intelligence community to rethink how it does its job. *NBC News*. Retrieved from www.nbcnews.com/politics/national-security/ coronavirus-may-force-u-s-intelligence-community-rethink-how-it-n1223811

Epstein, G. (2001). Controlling biological warfare threats: Resolving potential tensions among the research community, industry, and the national security community. *Critical Reviews in Microbiology*, *27*(4), 321–354.

Geissler, E. & Van Courtland Moon, J.E. (eds.). (1999). *Biological and Toxic Weapons: Research, Development, and Use from the Middle Ages to 1945*. Oxford, UK: Oxford University Press.

Gioe, D.V., Hatfield, J.M., & Stout, M. (2020). Can United States intelligence community analysts telework? *Intelligence and National Security*, *35*(6), 885–901. http://doi.org/ 10.1080/02684527.2020.1767389

Government of Canada, Canadian Security Intelligence Service (2022). Academic Outreach and Stakeholder Engagement. Retrieved from www.canada.ca/en/security-intelligence- service/corporate/academic-outreach.html

Guillemin, J. (1999). *Anthrax: The Investigation of a Deadly Outbreak*. Berkeley, CA: University of California Press.

Guillemin, J., Nowicke, J.W., Meselson, M., Akratanakul, P., & Seeley, T.D. (1985). Yellow rain. *Scientific American*.

Harris, S. (2021). CIA Creates New Mission Center to Counter China. *The Washington Post*. Retrieved from www.washingtonpost.com/national-security/cia-china-mission-cen ter/2021/10/06/fd477142-26d4-11ec-8d53-67cfb452aa60_story.html

Henderson, D.A., Inglesby, T.V., Bartlett, J.G., Ascher, M.S., Eitzen, E., Jahrling, P.B., Hauer, J., Layton, M., McDade, J., Osterholm, M.T., O'Toole, T., Parker, G., Perl, T., Russell, P.K., & Tonat, K. (1999). Smallpox as a biological weapon: Medical and public health management. *JAMA*, *281*(22), 2127–2137. http://doi.org/10.1001/jama.281.22.2127

Henricks, S.C. (2017). Social media, publicly available information, and the intelligence community. *American Intelligence Journal*, *34*(1), 21–31.

Intelligence Advanced Research Projects Agency (n.d.). *COVID-19 Research*. Retrieved from www.iarpa.gov/covid-19-research

Jehn, M., Pandit, U., Sabin, S., Tompkins, C., White, J., Kaleta, E., Dale, A.P., Ross, H.M., Kerr, R., Wolfe, T., Donegan, R., & Pappas, A. (2005). Collection and analysis on Iraq: Issues for the US. *Intelligence Community*, *49*(3), 47–54.

Koryakina, A. & Jolokhava, T. (2020). *Potential Corruption in Coronavirus-Related Public Tenders in Georgia*. Retrieved from www.bellingcat.com/news/rest-of-world/2020/07/ 31/corruption-in-coronavirus-related-public-tenders-in-georgia/

Landon-Murray, M. & Anderson, I. (2021). Making intelligence telework work: Mitigating distraction, maintaining focus. *Intelligence and National Security*, *36*(7), 1053–1056. https://doi.org/10.1080/02684527.2021.1955442

Lentzos, F., Goodman, M.S. & Wilson, J.M. (2020). Health Security Intelligence: Engaging across disciplines and sectors. *Intelligence and National Security*, *35*(4), 465–476. https://doi.org/10.1080/02684527.2020.1750166

Lentzos, F. & Littlewood, J. (2022). Russia finds another stage for the Ukraine biolabs disinformation show. *The Bulletin of the Atomic Scientists*. Retrieved from https://thebulletin.org/2022/07/russia-finds-another-stage-for-the-ukraine-biolabs-disinformation-show/

Ling, J. (2022). False claims of U.S. Biowarfare Labs in Ukraine Grip QAnon. *Foreign Policy*. Retrieved from https://foreignpolicy.com/2022/03/02/ukraine-biolabs-conspiracy-theory-qanon/

Marquardt, A. (2021). CIA will focus on China with new mission center. *CNN*. Retrieved from www.cnn.com/2021/10/07/politics/cia-china-mission-center/index.html

McCullough, J.M., Pepin, S., Kenny, K., Sanborn, H., Heywood, N., Schnall, A.H., Lant, T., & Sunenshine, R. (2022). Accuracy of case-based seroprevalence of SARS-CoV-2 antibodies in Maricopa County, Arizona. *American Journal of Public Health*, *112*(1), 38–42. https://doi.org/10.2105/AJPH.2021.306568

Morens, D.M., Breman, J.G., Calisher, C.H., Doherty, P.C., Hahn, B.H., Keusch, G.T., Kramer, L.D., Le Duc, J.W., Monath, T.P., & Taubenberger, J.K. (2020). The origin of COVID-19 and why it matters. *American Journal of Tropical Medicine and Hygiene*, *103*(3), 955–959.

National Intelligence Council (2021). *Global Trends 2040: A Contested World*. Retrieved from www.dni.gov/files/images/globalTrends/GT2040/GlobalTrends_2040_for_web1.pdf

National Science Foundation (2021). *New US-Canada Partnership Announced for Collaboration in Research and Innovation*. Retrieved from www.nsf.gov/news/special_reports/announcements/061521.jsp#:~:text=The%20U.S.%20National%20Science%20Foundation%20and%20the%20Natural,fundamental%20discovery%20research%20in%20the%20U.S.%20and%20Canada

National Science Foundation (2022). *SBE-UKRI Lead Agency Opportunity (SBE-UKRI)*. https://beta.nsf.gov/funding/opportunities/sbe-ukri-lead-agency-opportunity-sbe-ukri

Nemfakos, C. Rostker, B.D., Conley, R.E., Young, S., Williams, W.A., Engstrom, J., Bicksler, B., Elson, S.B., Jenkins, J., Kennedy-Boudali, L., & Temple, D. (2013). *Workforce Planning in the Intelligence Community*. Santa Monica, CA: RAND.

Office of National Intelligence (2023). *National Intelligence and Security Discovery Research Grants 2023 Round 3 Intelligence Challenges*. Retrieved from www.researchgrants.gov.au/sites/default/files/2022-07/NI23R1_Intelligence_Challenges.pdf

Office of Naval Research (n.d.). *Singapore*. Retrieved from www.nre.navy.mil/organization/onr-global/locations-global/singapore-onr-global

Office of the Director of National Intelligence (n.d.). *Intelligence Community Public-Private Talent Exchange*. Retrieved from https://www.dni.gov/index.php/careers/special-programs/ppte

Office of the Director of National Intelligence/National Intelligence Council (2021). *Updated Assessment on COVID-19 Origins*. Retrieved from www.odni.gov/files/ODNI/documents/assessments/Declassified-Assessment-on-COVID-19-Origins.pdf

Office of the Director of National Intelligence (2023). *Annual Threat Assessment of the U.S. Intelligence Community*. Retrieved from www.odni.gov/files/ODNI/documents/assessments/ATA-2023-Unclassified-Report.pdf

Pollard, S., & Kuznar, L. (2022). *A World Emerging from Pandemic*. Bethesda, MD: NI Press.

Richelson, J.T. (2015). Open sources site exploitation, and foreign materiel acquisition. In: Richelson, J.T. (ed.), *The US Intelligence Community*, 7th ed. New York: Routledge, 346–369.

Ross, H.M., Desiderio, S., St. Mars, T., & Rangel, P. (2021). US immigration policies pose a health security threat in COVID-19. *Health Security, 19*(S1), S83–S88. https://doi.org/10.1089/hs.2021.0039

Russell, R.L. (2007). *Sharpening Strategic Intelligence.* Cambridge, UK: Cambridge University Press.

Seth, S. (2018). *Difference and Disease: Medicine, Race, and the Eighteenth-Century British Empire.* Cambridge, UK: Cambridge University Press.

Smallman-Raynor, M.R. & Cliff, A.D. (2004). Impact of infectious diseases on war. *Infectious Disease Clinics of North America, 18*(2), 341–368. https://doi.org/10.1016/j.idc.2004.01.009

Smith, K.M., Machalaba, C.C., Seifman R., Feferholtz, Y., & Karesh W.B. (2019). Infectious disease and economics: The case for considering multi-sectoral impacts. *One Health, 7*(100080), 1–6. https://doi.org/10.1016/j.onehlt.2018.100080

Taylor, S. (2019). *The Psychology of Pandemics: Preparing for the Next Global Outbreak of Infectious Disease.* Newcastle upon Tyne, UK: Cambridge Scholars.

The Intelligence Community Inc. (n.d.). *Fellows Program.* Retrieved from www.theintell igencecommunity.com/internship-program/

Tian, E. (2020). *WHO Director-General Attacked on Twitter with CCP-Related Memes.* Retrieved from www.bellingcat.com/news/2020/08/21/who-director-general-attacked-on-twitter-with-ccp-related-memes/

Tiernan, J.-L. (2017). The practice of open intelligence: The experience of the canadian security intelligence service. In: Juneau, T. (ed.), *Strategic Analysis in Support of International Policy Making: Case Studies in Achieving Analytical Relevance.* United Kingdom: Rowman & Littlefield, 147–162.

Tilley, C. (2022). This is playing with fire – it could spark a lab-generated pandemic: Experts slam Boston lab where scientists have created a new deadly Omicron strain with an 80% kill rate in mice. *Daily Mail.* Retrieved from www.dailymail.co.uk/health/article-11323 677/Outrage-Boston-University-CREATES-Covid-strain-80-kill-rate.html

Torok, T.J., Tauxe, R.V., Wise, R.P., Livengood, J.R., Sokolow, R., & Mauvais, S. (1997). A large community outbreak of salmonellosis caused by intentional contamination of restaurant salad bars. *JAMA, 278*(5), 389–395.

UK Research and Innovation (2022). *International Agreements.* Retrieved from www.ukri.org/about-us/epsrc/relationships/international-agreements/lead-agency-opportun ity-with-the-nsf/

U.S. Department of State Bureau of Intelligence and Research (n.d.). *Analytic Exchanges.* Retrieved from www.state.gov/bureaus-offices/secretary-of-state/bureau-of-intelligence-and-research/

U.S. Embassy Singapore (2021). *Office of Naval Research Global (ONRG).* Retrieved from https://sg.usembassy.gov/office-of-naval-research-global-onrg/

U.S. National Academies of Science, Engineering, and Medicine (n.d.). *Jefferson Science Fellowship Program.* Retrieved from https://sites.nationalacademies.org/PGA/Jefferson/index.htm

Vogel, K.M. (2013). *Phantom Menace or Looming Danger?: A New Framework for Assessing Bioweapons Threats.* Baltimore, MD: The Johns Hopkins University Press.

Vogel, K.M. & Tyler, B.B. (2019). Interdisciplinary, cross-sector collaboration in the US intelligence community: Lessons learned from past and present efforts. *Intelligence and National Security, 34*(6), 851–880. https://doi.org/10.1080/02684527.2019.1620545

Walsh, P.F. (2016). *Submission to 2017 Independent Intelligence Review.* Retrieved from https://researchoutput.csu.edu.au/ws/portalfiles/portal/11937010/2016_Submission_to_Indep_Intel_Review_by_Walsh_21_Dec.pdf

Walsh, P.F. (2020). Improving 'five eyes' health security intelligence capabilities: leadership and governance challenges. *Intelligence and National Security*, *35*(4), 586–602. https://doi.org/10.1080/02684527.2020.1750156

Walsh, P.F. (2022). Email communication to author.

Wheelis, M. (2000). Investigating disease outbreaks under a protocol to the biological and toxin weapons convention. *Emerging Infectious Disease*, *6*(6), 595–600. https://doi.org/10.3201/eid0606.000607

Wilson, J.M. (2016). Signal recognition during the emergence of pandemic influenza type A/H1N1: A commercial disease intelligence unit's perspective. *Intelligence and National Security*, *32*(2), 222–230.

Wilson, J.M. (2018). The use of intelligence to determine attribution of the 2010 Haiti cholera disaster. *Intelligence and National Security*, *33*(6), 1–9.

Wilson, J.M., Lake, C.K., Matthews, M., Southard, M., Leone, R.M., & McCarthy, M. (2022). Health security warning intelligence during first contact with COVID: an operations perspective. *Intelligence and National Security*, *37*(2), 216–240. doi: 10.1080/02684527.2021.2020034

Wilson, J.M. & McNamara, T. (2020). The 1999 West Nile virus warning signal revisited. *Intelligence and National Security*, *35*(4), 519–526. doi: 10.1080/02684527.2020.1750144

Winter, H., Gerster, L., Helmer, J., & Baaken, T. (2021). *Disinformation Overdose: A Study of the Crisis of Trust Among Vaccine Sceptics and Anti Vaxers*. Berlin, Germany: Institute for Strategic Dialogue. Retrieved from www.isdglobal.org/wp-content/uploads/2021/07/Disinformation-Overdose3.pdf

World Health Organization (n.d.). *WHO Collaborating Center for Global Health Security*. Retrieved from https://apps.who.int/whocc/Detail.aspx?5vYG8fmWM7yT6erZjSEr8w==

9 Managing Health Security Threats at the Multilateral Level

The Challenge of Investigating Ambiguous Outbreaks

Filippa Lentzos

Introduction

At the international level, the World Health Organization (WHO) has traditionally played a central role in alerting states and communities to developing disease outbreaks and in supporting national and international responses. The COVID-19 pandemic was no exception. On 31 December 2019, the WHO Country Office in China picked up a media statement on the Wuhan Municipal Health Commission website reporting cases of "viral pneumonia" in Wuhan. The Country Office notified the International Health Regulations (IHR) focal point in the WHO Western Pacific Regional Office about the media statement. On the same day, the WHO's Epidemic Intelligence from Open Sources (EIOS) platform also picked up a media report on ProMED (a programme of the International Society for Infectious Diseases) about the same cluster of cases in Wuhan. Several health authorities from around the world also reported information on the cluster of atypical pneumonia cases from the Chinese authorities. On 2 January 2020, the WHO Representative in China wrote to the National Health Commission of China, offering WHO support and repeating the request for further information on the cluster of cases. The WHO also informed its sister United Nations (UN) agencies, international organizations, major public health agencies and laboratories, which are all part of its Global Outbreak Alert and Response Network (GOARN), about the atypical pneumonia cases, which later became named COVID-19.

The WHO also played a central role, as it has in past epidemics and pandemics, of investigating the origins of COVID-19. But the investigation—and the political controversy that ensued and that continues to plague the investigation—highlighted a significant gap in the international community's ability to investigate outbreaks where it is not clear whether the outbreak results from natural, accidental or deliberate causes.

These ambiguous events are likely to become more frequent in future. Risks of natural outbreaks from zoonotic transmissions are increasing for a host of reasons including human population growth and our continued encroachment on animal habitats as well as intensive farming and wildlife trade. Climate change, too, is a factor, not only increasing the frequency of interactions with animals but also altering vector distribution, leading to the emergence of tick- and mosquito-borne

DOI: 10.4324/9781003335511-12

infections in regions where they were previously uncommon. The risks of laboratory accidents are increasing as more high containment laboratories are built around
the world and ever more extreme high-risk experiments are conducted, including
so-called "gain-of-function" research that enhances the virulence or transmissibility of potential pandemic pathogens compared to naturally occurring strains.
Growth in large-scale viral prospecting and more intense field sampling are also
contributing to accidental outbreaks from research-related activities. Finally, risks
of deliberate outbreaks are increasing as barriers to developing biological weapons
are coming down and advances in science and technology mean that it is technic-
ally possible for biological weapons to emerge that are capable of causing greater
harm than before, that are more accessible to more people, with attacks that can be
more precisely targeted, and that can be harder to attribute.

While the WHO has traditionally taken the lead on investigating naturally-
occurring outbreaks, the UN General Assembly has bestowed the UN Secretary-
General with powers to investigate allegations of deliberately-caused outbreaks.
Moreover, the Biological and Toxin Weapons Convention (BWC) provides its 185
states parties with the ability to request that the UN Security Council investigate an
allegation of biological weapons use, and the Security Council can also establish
an investigation outside of the BWC as it did with the UN Special Commission
on Iraq (UNSCOM). However, while both the health and security spheres have
mechanisms in place for investigation, there are no agreed multilateral processes
for investigating accidentally caused outbreaks.

As an outbreak unfolds, it might not be clear whether it is naturally, accidentally
or deliberately caused. A key challenge for the international community highlighted
by the COVID-19 pandemic is how to effectively investigate outbreak origins
while remaining open to all three possibilities. This chapter details COVID-19
origin investigations in 2020, 2021 and 2022; sets out three proposals currently on
the table to address the investigation gap; and, rejecting these proposals, provides
a more near-term and pragmatic alternative for how the international community
should handle investigations into outbreaks of ambiguous origins.

Investigating the Origins of COVID-19

The WHO's first novel coronavirus press conference on 14 January 2020
highlighted the importance of finding the animal source of SARS-CoV-2 (World
Health Organization [WHO] 2020a). The first IHR Emergency Committee of independent scientific experts advising the WHO Director-General, Tedros Adhanom
Ghebreyesus, on the pandemic recommended convening an international multi-
disciplinary mission, including national experts, to "review and support efforts
to investigate the animal source of the outbreak" (WHO 2020b). The Director-
General directly raised the matter of identifying the virus origins and intermediate
hosts with President Xi Jinping during his visit to China in January 2020 (WHO
2020c).

While not its main focus, considering the source of SARS-CoV-2 formed part
of the WHO–China Joint Mission in February 2020. Led by a senior adviser to

the WHO director-general and the chief expert of the Chinese National Health Commission, the mission team comprised 25 experts from the WHO, China, Germany, Japan, Republic of Korea, Nigeria, Russia, Singapore and the USA (Mallapaty 2020). Over nine days beginning on 16 February, the mission team consulted provincial governors, municipal mayors, senior scientists, public health workers and others. They visited hospitals, disease control agencies, transport hubs and emergency supply warehouses in Beijing, Guangdong and Sichuan. They also visited a wet market, though not the one in Wuhan that had been identified as the possible spillover site. Only select team members travelled to Wuhan, where they visited a hospital and a mobile cabin hospital. The mission report concluded that the novel coronavirus was a zoonotic virus, that bats appeared to be the virus reservoir, and that no intermediate hosts had yet been identified (WHO China Joint Mission 2020). One of the report's recommendations was that "additional effort should be made to find the animal source, including the natural reservoir and any intermediate amplification host, to prevent any new epidemic foci or resurgence of similar epidemics" (WHO 2020c). To that end, and in line with the prevailing theory that the spillover event happened at a wet market, the mission report highlighted activities already underway by Chinese authorities to investigate the pandemic's origins. These involved taking environmental samples from the Huanan Wholesale Seafood Market in Wuhan and obtaining records about the wildlife species sold at the market, as well as examining early COVID-19 cases in Wuhan (WHO China Joint Mission 2020).

The joint mission's call for greater efforts to examine the pandemic's origins was later echoed by the IHR Emergency Committee on the pandemic. Ahead of the annual May meeting of the World Health Assembly, the group advised the WHO to "work with the World Organisation for Animal Health (OIE), the Food and Agriculture Organization of the United Nations (FAO), and countries to identify the zoonotic source of the virus and the route of introduction to the human population, including the possible role of intermediate hosts" (WHO China Joint Mission 2020). In the days before the World Health Assembly meeting, the European Union (EU), Australia and others also called for an international investigation into the origins of the pandemic (Lentzos 2020).

At the opening of the virtual meeting of the 73rd World Health Assembly on 18–19 May 2020, President Xi Jinping, who had previously strongly opposed an international investigation, seemed to reverse his stance and support an international review—albeit a review on his own terms (Niquet 2020). The World Health Assembly's resolution on the COVID-19 response echoed the IHR Emergency Committee's request to the WHO Director-General "to continue to work closely" with the OIE, the FAO and states on identifying the virus's zoonotic source and path of transmission to humans, "as part of the One-Health Approach," "including through efforts such as scientific and collaborative field missions" (World Health Assembly 2020).

Based on the request, the WHO and China began work to initiate "a series of studies that will contribute to origin tracing work" (WHO 2021a). In July, WHO experts travelled to China to define the role of the international investigative team, which was to explore the potential sources of infection amongst the first reported cases in Wuhan in December 2019, to attempt to identify earlier human cases through sero-epidemiologic studies, and to conduct further animal and environmental studies (WHO 2021d). The investigative team, agreed by both the WHO and China, was formed in September, but only made public on 20 November 2020. The team included a broad range of expertise with experts from Australia, Denmark, Germany, Japan, the Netherlands, Russia, the UK, the USA, Vietnam and Qatar, and also included five WHO experts, two FAO representatives and two OIE representatives—alongside an equal number of scientists (17) from China (WHO 2020c). The first virtual meeting of the international experts with their Chinese counterparts was held on 30 October 2020, (WHO 2020c) and the terms of reference for the Global Study of the Origins of SARS-CoV-2 was published on 5 November 2020 (WHO 2021b).

The terms of reference show clear indications of a political settlement between the WHO and China. They emphasized that "the virus may have circulated elsewhere" before it was "identified through surveillance in Wuhan" and that "the global origin tracing work is therefore not bound to any location and may evolve geographically as evidence is being generated, and hypotheses evolve" (WHO 2021c). The document is firmly in line with Beijing's origins narrative from the second half of 2020 that SARS-CoV-2 may have initially spilled over in Italy, France, the United States, or elsewhere and circulated undetected before it was identified in Wuhan, or that the virus may have been introduced to China through imported food products. The terms of reference note that there is currently no evidence of SARS-CoV-2 transmission on food products, but the document stresses, on multiple occasions, the possibility of an origin outside China (WHO 2021c).

The joint WHO–China team, plagued by delays, finally began its field visit to China in January 2021. In advance of it doing so, and very late in its tenure, the outgoing US Trump administration issued a fact sheet on the pandemic's origins on 15 January 2021 (US Department of State 2021). It said SARS-CoV-2 could have first entered the human population through human contact with infected animals. Alternatively, it could have spilled over into the human population as a result of a lab accident, where "initial exposure included only a few individuals and was compounded by asymptomatic infection." The fact sheet noted that "scientists in China have researched animal-derived coronaviruses under conditions that increased the risk for accidental and potentially unwitting exposure," and listed three elements deserving "greater scrutiny." All associated with the Wuhan Institute of Virology (the premier laboratory in China working on coronaviruses), these three elements were genetic experiments with coronaviruses, COVID-19-like illnesses in the autumn of 2019 and secret military activity at the institute. The US fact sheet said that "any credible investigation into the origin of COVID-19 demands complete, transparent access to the research labs in Wuhan, including their facilities, samples, personnel, and records" (US Department of State 2021).

After four weeks of work, including two weeks of quarantine imposed on the international experts by the Chinese government, the joint WHO–China mission reported its highly anticipated findings at a press conference on 9 February 2021 in

Wuhan (WHO 2021e). The co-heads of the mission, Peter Ben Embarek and Liang Wannian, laid out four origin hypotheses that had formed the basis of the mission's investigation. First, the virus could have jumped directly from an animal species to humans. Alternatively, and second, the virus could have leapt from one animal species to an intermediary animal host in which the virus further adapted before jumping to people. A third, and surprising, hypothesis, which had not featured in prior origin discussions, was that the virus could have been introduced to Wuhan via the food chain, for example from imported frozen products. A final hypothesis was that the virus could have been accidentally released through a lab-related incident. The joint mission, made up of Chinese scientists selected by China and an equal number of international experts selected by the WHO, concluded that the second hypothesis, where the virus jumped from one species to another before infecting people, was the "most likely" pathway (WHO 2021). While the mission reported that the direct spill over and food-chain ideas needed more investigation, Ben Embarek said the team dismissed the lab-leak hypothesis as "extremely unlikely" and that it would not be pursued any further.

Although the findings of the joint team were widely reported in the press as representing the findings of the WHO itself, they did not represent the official position of the WHO. This was made clear two days after the press conference briefing, when the WHO Director-General undercut the remarks by Ben Embarek and the team, by "clarifying" that no hypotheses had been ruled out and that "all hypotheses remain open and require further study" (WHO 2021d).

The mission report was eventually released on 30 March 2021, seven weeks after the mission ended (WHO 2021). It showed that the joint team saw its priority as seeking a zoonotic origin, not as fully examining all possible sources of the pandemic. The published data supporting the report mostly presented reviews of Chinese studies that had not been published, shared with, or reviewed by the international scientific community. The report also showed that, well over a year after the initial outbreak, critical records and biological samples that could have provided essential insights into the pandemic origins remained inaccessible and had not been accessed by the team. The international members of the joint team, by their own admission, had often relied on verbal assurances given to them by their Chinese counterparts rather than independent investigation. This was particularly the case when it came to the possibility of a research-related accident. The final process used by the joint team for assessing the likelihoods of a natural spillover or a research-related accident—amounting to a show of hands by the team members based on a superficial review—failed to reach basic standards of credible analysis and assessment. The report also showed that it was, at best, unclear whether the Chinese team members had the leeway to express their fair evaluation of the origin theories in the presence of their Chinese government minders. Finally, the report made clear that the team had used different evidentiary standards for the origin theories it assessed.

On the day the report came out, the WHO Director-General further distanced himself and the WHO from the team's findings. In a statement, he said that all origin hypotheses must still be examined, including the possibility of a lab-related incident; that China must be more forthright in sharing essential data and bio-logical samples; and that the WHO was prepared to send additional missions and experts to China to thoroughly examine all origin hypotheses (WHO 2021). A joint statement, on the same day, by 14 countries, led by the United States, was also critical of the report (US Department of State 2021). It underscored the need for a transparent and independent analysis, free from interference and undue influence, and it voiced the countries' shared concern that the joint study lacked access to complete, original data and samples. A similar statement was made by the European Union (European Union 2021). Independent experts also voiced concern about the joint mission's independence, investigation process and conclusions (New York Times 2021).

On 13 May 2021, 18 leading scientists published a letter in the prestigious journal *Science* calling for a full investigation into all pandemic origin hypoth-esis, including a lab incident (Bloom et al. 2021). This followed an earlier open letter on 4 March from scientists and social scientists calling for a full investigation into the pandemic's origins (Butler et al. 2021). On 26 May 2021, President Biden issued a statement saying he had asked the US intelligence community to inves-tigate the origin question and to report back to the White House in 90 days (The White House 2021a). Over the course of the spring and early summer of 2021, the lab-leak theory was also given greater prominence in the media (Wade 2021; Jacobsen 2021; Eban 2021).

A 13 June 2021 statement by G7 leaders meeting in Cornwall, England stressed that the second phase of the WHO-convened origins study should take place in China and be "timely, transparent, expert-led, and science-based" (The White House 2021b, para. 16). At a press briefing on 15 July 2021, the WHO Director-General told reporters that for the second phase of the origins study the WHO was "asking China to be transparent, open and cooperate, especially on the informa-tion, raw data that we asked for at the early days of the pandemic" (WHO 2021). The Director-General expressed his view that there had been a "premature push" to rule out the lab theory, saying, "I was a lab technician myself, an immunologist, and I have worked in the lab, and lab accidents happen. It's common." In opening remarks to the "WHO member state information session on pandemic origins" on 16 July 2021, the WHO Director-General made clear operational plans and terms of reference for the second phase were still in development. He highlighted that the origins study "is a scientific exercise that must be kept free from politics" (WHO 2021). He continued: "For that to happen, we expect China to support this next phase of the scientific process by sharing all relevant data in a spirit of transpar-ency. Equally, we expect all member states to support the scientific process by refraining from politicising it" (WHO 2021d).

At the member state information session, the Director-General also announced that the WHO was establishing a permanent international scientific advisory group for origins of novel pathogens (SAGO), which would "play a vital role in the next phase of studies into the origins of SARS-CoV-2" (WHO 2021). The group even-tually selected comprised 27 individuals, including several scientists from the pre-vious joint WHO–China study (WHO 2021).

On 24 August 2021, the US intelligence community delivered its classified report on pandemic origins to President Biden, and a short, two-page unclassified summary was released on 27 August 2021 (Office of the Director of National Intelligence [ODNI] 2021). Made up of several agencies, the intelligence community was divided on the origin question. Four agencies and the National Intelligence Council assessed with low confidence that the pandemic was most likely caused by natural spillover. One agency assessed with moderate confidence that it was caused by a laboratory-associated incident. Three institutions were unable to make a judgment either way. These different assessments resulted from "how agencies weigh intelligence reporting and scientific publications, and intelligence and scientific gaps" (ODNI, 2021, para. 2). To reach a conclusive assessment the report said China's cooperation would most likely be needed. There were, however, two things the intelligence agencies could agree on. The first was that the virus was not developed as a biological weapon, and the second that the Chinese government did not have foreknowledge of the virus before the outbreak began. Most agencies also assessed, with low confidence, that SARS-CoV-2 was probably not genetically engineered, though two agencies believed there was insufficient evidence to make that judgement. On the release of the report, President Biden said that while the review had concluded, "our efforts to understand the origins of this pandemic will not rest" (The White House 2021c, para. 1). He stressed that "critical information about the origins of this pandemic exists in the People's Republic of China, yet from the beginning, government officials in China have worked to prevent international investigators and members of the global public health community from accessing it" (The White House 2021c, para. 2). He said the United States would continue to press China to fully share information and to cooperate with the WHO's second phase of the origins study. He concluded that "we must have a full and transparent accounting of this global tragedy. Nothing less is acceptable" (The White House 2021c, para. 3).

In June 2022, the WHO released the first preliminary report from the scientific advisory group for the origins of novel pathogens (WHO 2022). The report noted that no new data had been made available to evaluate the 'lab leak' hypothesis and recommended further investigations on origins. It recognized that lab leaks had happened historically with other pathogens, and that it was important to include studies to address risks of biosafety or biosecurity breaches. The report provided key recommendations "for further studies needed on humans, animals and the environment in China and around the world" (WHO 2022, 5). The SAGO emphasized the preliminary nature of the report, and that work was ongoing, but indicated that "currently available epidemiological and sequencing data suggest ancestral strains to SARS-CoV-2 have a zoonotic origin" (WHO 2022, 5). However, the SAGO also noted that it would "remain open to any and all scientific evidence that becomes available in the future to allow for comprehensive testing of all reasonable hypotheses" (WHO 2022, 6).

Nevertheless, the lab leak theory continues to be a source of political tension. In response to the SAGO's preliminary report, the Chinese Ministry of Foreign Affairs reverted to its defensive narrative that the origins study must be conducted "on the basis of science and free from political interference" (Chinese Ministry of

Foreign Affairs 2022). It continued: "The lab leak theory is a false claim concocted by anti-China forces for political purposes. It has nothing to do with science. The Chinese side has invited WHO experts to visit the Wuhan lab, and the joint report reached the clear conclusion that 'a laboratory origin of the pandemic was considered to be extremely unlikely'. Since the SAGO report has called for investigation into biological laboratories 'located worldwide where early COVID-19 cases have been retrospectively detected' for the next phase of study, investigation should first target highly suspicious laboratories such as those at Fort Detrick and the University of North Carolina in the US" (Chinese Ministry of Foreign Affairs 2022). In October 2022 a US Senate committee released its own interim report on the origins of the pandemic, which concluded that "the Covid-19 pandemic was, more likely than not, the result of a research-related incident" (US Senate Committee on Health, Education, Labor and Pensions 2022, 26).

There are many lessons that can be taken away from the COVID-19 origins investigation. Three overriding ones are: (1) a mandate and process for investigating an ambiguous outbreak needs to be in place *before* the outbreak happens; it cannot be negotiated as it unfolds; (2) established rules and procedures of operation, covering, among other things, sample collection and access to people, institutions, records, databases and documents, must be agreed in advance; and (3) an origin investigation of an ambiguous outbreak must have in-built capacity to go beyond a standard epidemiological investigation and switch to a forensic mode of investigation if required (Lentzos 2020).

Proposals for New International Investigative Powers

The need to establish an investigative body, residing at the nexus between the public health and security spheres, was apparent to some already before the World Health Assembly agreed on collaborative field missions to identify the origins of SARS-CoV-2 in May 2020. The former British foreign secretary, Lord William Hague of Richmond, for example, declared that animal to human virus transmission must in future be treated as a weapon of mass destruction, and, just as the world has systems to monitor nuclear facilities and ban the proliferation of weapons of mass destruction, so too, Hague said, it is time for a new international order to inspect the biological threats that "pose the greatest danger to human health and the global economy" (Wright 2020). Hague was speaking at the launch of a report by the conservative think tank Policy Exchange which called for "a new or strengthened co-ordinating body at the international level, ideally UN-based, to lead the monitoring, research and inspection of high-risk activities" that increase risks of zoonotic disease outbreaks (Policy Exchange 2020).

The idea of a new international body that could inspect high-risk activities and investigate outbreaks of unknown origin have also been raised by others. One key initiative, whose impetus, among other things, were the "numerous suspicions and accusations that the COVID-19 virus was man-made, that the pandemic leaked from a laboratory or was part of a biological weapons program," calls for an International Agency for Biological Safety and was first introduced by the

President of Kazakhstan, Kassym-Jomart Tokayev, to the UN General Assembly in October 2020 (Biological and Toxin Weapons Convention [BWC] 2020, para. 4). Framed within the Biological and Toxin Weapons Convention (BWC), and further elaborated at the ninth review conference of BWC in 2022, the proposal envisages a range of functions for the agency including the power to conduct inspections of biological activities as well as a rapid response team of permanently employed and trained experts to be dispatched in case of accidental or deliberate use of bioweapons on the request of the state concerned (BWC 2022).

A second initiative calls for a new Joint Assessment Mechanism (JAM) "to rapidly identify the origins of high-consequence biological events, specifically in cases where there is ambiguity about whether an outbreak is naturally emerging or the result of a deliberate or accidental release" (Kane et al. 2022). Proposed by the Nuclear Threat Initiative (NTI), it envisages an internationally diverse roster of scientific experts within the office of the UN Secretary-General that would conduct ongoing data analysis and that would have "an operational capability to rapidly launch an assessment of a biological event of unknown origin—within 48 hours of UN authorization." "Its mandate would be to establish the facts regarding the origin of an unusual outbreak, and its approach would be rapid, transparent, and evidence-based," taking advantage of new tools, methods and technologies, such as bioinformatics, data science and AI, and building on existing resources associated with existing UN investigative mechanisms.

Regardless of their merits, proposals to establish new multilaterally agreed bodies or mechanisms simply do not match today's political reality. While they can be goals for the longer term, more immediate near-term solutions are needed. A public health-focused, rather than security-focused, investigation mechanism is likely the most politically palatable approach to a state where an outbreak starts spreading—and cooperation from the origin state would be crucial for an effective investigation as the COVID-19 investigation has demonstrated. Any measures introduced have a higher chance of acceptance if they are anchored in existing international frameworks and are as minimally intrusive as possible. The WHO, as the world's premier forum for dealing with public health and with a global on-the-ground presence, is an obvious choice, and while politicized, it is fairly science-driven, and certainly less politicized than other international forums like the UN General Assembly, the UN Human Rights Council, or the UN Security Council, where one country or another frequently blocks international action on a given issue seemingly as a matter of course. Going through the WHO also means all member states would contribute, and have a stake in, an investigation through funding from assessed contributions. The WHO's existing International Health Regulations provide a clear mechanism for expansion to enable a stepwise methodology to guide an ambiguous origin investigation.

A Pragmatic Approach to Investigating Outbreaks with Ambiguous Origins

Any ambiguous origin investigation should start from an initial focus on natural origin sources and build on traditional epidemiological principles. The investigation would typically begin with defining the *Who, What, When, and Where* of infection. Investigators would take case histories and conduct interviews to determine who is being infected, by what disease agent, when infection occurred, and in what location. By first describing the epidemiology in this way, investigators can ask the following key questions to explore potential indicators of a laboratory accident or unusual source: Is the infecting agent unusual for the location, or time of year? And, is it affecting unusual populations, in unusual ways?

Next, investigators would seek to determine the *How* and *Why* of infection. How did infection occur, and what circumstances enabled infection? To explore these analytical epidemiology questions, investigators typically assess, first, the epidemiological triangle (the relationship between a disease agent (typically in an animal reservoir), a human host and the environment) for indicators of convergence that would enable spillover of the infecting agent from its natural reservoir to humans. If no epidemiological link is apparent, investigators can seek to identify risk factors that might enable such exposure by asking the following key questions: Has the human population expanded into areas where the disease agent resides in animal reservoirs, for example due to wildlife trade, deforestation, or industrial farming? Has the disease agent expanded into human populations, for example due to animal reservoir overgrowth, vector population overgrowth (e.g., ticks, fleas), or interspecies spillover? Has the environment brought animal and human populations closer together, for example due to short-term meteorological shifts or longer-term climate shifts? To continue the exploration of the *How* and *Why*, investigators would assess the infecting agent genome for indicators of geographical and temporal spread. By comparing the infecting agent's genome with the genomes of well-characterized reference strains in the public domain, investigators can identify the closest known relative of the infecting agent and determine whether the infecting agent's genome has amassed mutations consistent with known patterns of natural emergence. For example, SARS-CoV-2's genome closely resembles that of a bat coronavirus (Zhou et al. 2020) but a small section of the genome called the "polybasic cleavage site," believed to provide a selective advantage for disease transmission, would have been expected to evolve over time but instead is present in the earliest sequences of the virus Zhan et al. 2020). Investigators can further determine whether the infecting agent's genome so closely resembles a given reference strain that a period of limited or no replication is likely. Such so-called "frozen evolution," when an infecting agent's genome lacks the expected accumulation of mutations over time, suggests that alternate origin hypotheses such as a laboratory accident must be explored (Pascall et al. 2020).

Based on descriptive and analytical epidemiology findings, investigators may collect and/or analyze additional animal, human or environmental samples with the goal of closing information gaps in the prevailing origin hypothesis. If contact with an animal reservoir is suspected, investigators may collect animal or environmental samples at the suspected animal–human interface, whether a market, farm, abattoir, or in the wild. Analysis of these samples may identify the reservoir or provide additional clues that can be traced back epidemiologically and genetically. "Banked" human samples predating the outbreak may also be tested to this end; often, such clinical samples are retained for extended periods of time, and may be revisited for further analysis, for example if they came from patients with clinical presentations resembling the current outbreak (Deslandes et al. 2020). In addition, investigators may actively collect human samples that might indicate exposure or infection in so-called sentinel populations at the animal–human interface. For example, serological testing of hunters or wildlife traders may identify antibodies against the agent causing the current outbreak, indicating exposure that may then be traced back to an animal reservoir (Dovih et al. 2019). If a natural source is not identified, or if early evidence indicates a potential laboratory source, the search for a natural source should continue as the investigation expands to include laboratory sources. At this point, unrestricted access to need-to-know information, site and personnel becomes increasingly necessary.

If expansion of the investigation to include potential laboratory sources is warranted, the first step is to perform a risk assessment of proximal laboratories to identify: what biological agents or unknown/suspect samples are being worked with that might be relevant to the outbreak (causing similar symptoms and signs, related genetically, or otherwise associated by person, place or time); using what techniques, such as high risk culturing (liquid bacterial culture or viral culture), animal studies, or genetic manipulation of relevant samples or specimens identified in the previous step; and at what level of biosafety to identify unsafe or uncertain safety conditions where high risk activities with relevant samples or specimens are being performed (Piltch & Pomper 2020). These factors determine the potential risk to surrounding communities that a laboratory mishap may spark an outbreak, for example due to worker infection, incomplete decontamination of waste, or aerosol release. Any combination of factors that poses undue or unknown risk to the surrounding community should be categorized as "high risk" requiring mitigation.

If the laboratory risk assessment indicates that further investigation is warranted—for example, relevant specimens or samples are present, high-risk activities are being performed, or safe working conditions are either lacking or uncertain—the next step is to perform a comprehensive onsite assessment. The assessment would require unrestricted access to the laboratory and its personnel, conditional upon the findings of the laboratory risk assessment.

To enable this stepwise methodology the current WHO's International Health Regulations would need to be expanded to cover an international investigative body with a mandate to enable need-to-know access to, at minimum, laboratory sample receiving and accessioning logs, and laboratory safety and security records, as well as conditional access to the laboratory and its personnel.

If findings at any stage of the outbreak investigation suggest the possibility of a deliberate origin, systematic sample collection, careful documentation of chain-of-custody to ensure the integrity of evidence, and analysis in accredited laboratories become paramount. Law enforcement must become involved either at the national level, possibly with support from other states, but most likely at the international level under the UN Secretary-General's Mechanism (UNSGM), and likely in coordination with other relevant international organizations such as the WHO, the World Organization for Animal Health (OIE, now WOAH) and Interpol. A security-focused investigation would involve additional evidence collection and examination, patient and witness interviews, coordination with intelligence officials regarding adversary capabilities and motivations, and targeted intelligence-gathering activities.

The mandate of the UNSGM, established by a General Assembly resolution in 1987, authorizes the Secretary-General to carry out an investigation into the possible use of chemical or biological weapons, including dispatching a fact-finding team to the site(s) of the alleged incident(s) (UNODA n.d). The Secretary-General is to promptly report the results of any such investigations to all member states. The UNSGM mandate was reaffirmed by the UN Security Council in 1988. Agreed guideline and procedures for a UNSGM investigation were endorsed by the General Assembly in 1990 and technical appendices were updated in 2007. The UNSGM is not a standing investigative body. Instead, member states nominate expert consultants, qualified experts and analytical laboratories which are then listed in a roster and may be called upon to support a UNSGM investigation. As of 30 December 2022, there were 562 qualified experts, 60 expert consultants and 88 analytical laboratories nominated by member states from all UN regions listed on the roster United Nations Office for Disarmament Affairs 2022).

There have, to date, not been any allegations of biological incidents, but UNSGM investigations have taken place for alleged use of chemical weapons in Mozambique and Azerbaijan in 1992 and in Syria in 2013. In addition, training activities provide UNSGM rostered experts with additional knowledge and skills to operate as a cohesive UN team in the challenging field conditions to carry out their mandate. The first training course was offered by Sweden in 2009, and, since then, more than 20 training courses have been held in six countries (Australia, Denmark, France, Germany, Sweden and the United Kingdom) as well as organized by two international organizations (INTERPOL and the Organisation for the Prohibition of Chemical Weapons). The most recent was the two-part Capstone exercise conducted by the Robert Koch Institute in Germany and completed in 2022, which involved a table-top exercise and a full-scale field exercise simulating an entire investigation mission of a deliberate biological outbreak.

Key next steps once the International Health Regulations have been expanded to include an international investigative body is to develop agreed guidelines and procedures, nominate rostered experts, and train them to investigate ambiguous events and to work collaboratively with UNSGM rostered experts.

Conclusion

Since COVID-19, the war in Ukraine, the assault on laboratories during Sudan's civil unrest, and earthquakes and floods in Syria, Morocco and Libya, have highlighted the precarity of biological security amidst the pressing concerns of conflict, climate change and natural disasters. With increasingly confrontative global geopolitics and active disinformation campaigns, future unusual disease outbreaks will likely have increased ambiguity about their origins. Suspicions and allegations about biological weapons are likely to become more frequent. Trends to this effect are already visible; for example, in allegations of BWC non-compliance and in disinformation campaigns on prohibited biological weapons-related activities, which have been a topic of formal consultations at the United Nations in Geneva.

To effectively investigate unusual disease outbreaks, it is crucial that the international community develops a mechanism that is open to possibilities of natural, accidental or deliberate origins. This chapter has set out a near-term and pragmatic proposal for how the international community could handle such an investigation.

References

73rd World Health Assembly (2020). *COVID-19 Response.* https://apps.who.int/gb/ebwha/pdf_files/WHA73/A73_R1-en.pdf

Biological Weapons Convention (2022, December 14). *Compliance by States Parties with All Their Obligations Under the Convention* [Background Information Submitted by the Implementation Support Unit]. https://disarmament.unoda.org/biological-weapons

Bloom, J. D., Chan, Y. A., Baric, R. S., Bjorkman, P. J., Cobey, S., Deverman, B. E., Fisman, D. N., Gupta, R., Iwasaki, A., Lipsitch, M., Medhitov, R., Neher, R. A., Nielsen, R., Patterson, N., Stearns, T., Nimwegen, E. V., Worobey, M., & Relman, D. A. (2021). Investigate the origins of COVID-19. *Science, 372*(6543). www.science.org/doi/10.1126/science.abj0016#tab-contributors

Butler et al. (2021). *Call for a Full and Unrestricted International Forensic Investigation into the Origins of COVID-19* [Open Letter]. New York Times. https://s.wsj.net/public/resources/documents/COVID%20OPEN%20LETTER%20FINAL%20030421%20(1).pdf; https://int.nyt.com/data/documenttools/virus-inquiries-pandemic-origins/d7a097a4c758a65a/full.pdf

Chinese Ministry of Foreign Affairs (2022). *Foreign Ministry Spokesperson Zhao Lijian's Regular Press Conference*, English Transcript, 10 June 2022. http://mz.china-embassy.gov.cn/por/fyrth/202206/t20220610_10701735.htm

Deslandes, A., Berti, V., Tandjoui-Lambotte, Y., Alloui, C., Carbonnelle, E., Zahar, J. R., Brichler, S., & Cohen Y. (2020). SARS-CoV-2 was already spreading in France in late December 2019. *International Journal of Antimicrobial Agents, 55*(6). https://doi.org/10.1016/j.ijantimicag.2020.106006

Dovih, P., Laing, E. D., Chen, Y., Low, D. H. W., Ansil, B. R., Yang, X., Shi, Z., Broder, C. C., Smith, G. J. D., Linster, M. N., Ramakrishnan, U., & Mendenhall, I. H. (2019). Filovirus-reactive antibodies in humans and bats in Northeast India imply zoonotic spill over. *PLoS Neglected Tropical Diseases, 13*(10). https://doi.org/10.1371/journal.pntd.000773

Eban, K. (2021, June 3). The lab-leak theory: Inside the fight to uncover COVID-19's origins. *Vanity Fair.* www.whitehouse.gov/briefing-room/statements-releases/2021/06/13/carbis-bay-g7-summit-communique/

European Union (2021, March 30). *EU Statement on the WHO-led COVID-19 Origins Study* [Statement]. https://eeas.europa.eu/delegations/un-geneva/95960/eu-statement-who-led-covid-19-origins-study_en

Jacobsen, R. (2021, February 6). Exclusive: How Amateur Sleuths Broke the Wuhan Lab Story and Embarrassed the Media. *Newsweek Magazine.* www.newsweek.com/exclusive-how-amateur-sleuths-broke-wuhan-lab-story-embarrassed-media-1596958

Kane, A., Yassif, J. M., Isaac, C., & Korol, S. (2022, April 25). Joint Assessment Mechanism to Determine Pandemic Origins. *Nuclear Threat Initiative.* www.nti.org/about/programs-projects/project/joint-assessment-mechanism-to-determine-pandemic-origins/

Lentzos, F. (2020, May 18). Will the WHO call for an international investigation into the coronavirus's origins? *Bulletin of Atomic Scientists.* https://thebulletin.org/2020/05/will-the-who-call-for-an-international-investigation-into-the-coronaviruss-origins

Mallapaty, S. (2020). The scientists investigating the pandemic's origins. *Nature.* *588*(208).

Niquet, V. (2020, May 19). Decoding Xi Jingping's speech at the World Health Assembly. *The Diplomat.* https://thediplomat.com/2020/05/decoding-xi-jinpings-speech-at-the-world-health-assembly/

Office of the Director of National Intelligence (2021.). *Unclassified Summary of Assessment on COVID-19 Origins.* www.dni.gov/files/ODNI/documents/assessments/Unclassified-Summary-of-Assessment-on-COVID-19-Origins.pdf

Pascall, D. J., Nomikou, K., Bréard, E., Zientara, S., da Silva Filipe, A., Hoffman, B., Jacquot, M., Singer, J. B., De Clercq, K., Bøtner, A., Sailleau, C., Viarouge, C., Batten, C., Puggioni, G., Ligos, C., Savini, G., van Rign, P. P. C., Biek, R., & Palmarini, M. (2020). "Frozen evolution" of an RNA virus suggests accidental release as a potential cause of arbovirus re-emergence. *PLoS Biology*, *18*(4). https://doi.org/10.1371/journal.pbio.3000673

Pilch, R. & Pomper, M. (2020). A guide to getting serious about bio-lab safety. *War on the Rocks.* https://warontherocks.com/2020/06/a-guide-to-getting-serious-about-bio-lab-safety/

The White House (2021a, June 13). *Carbis Bay G7 Summit Communiqué.* www.whitehouse.gov/briefing-room/statements-releases/2021/06/13/carbis-bay-g7-summit-communique/

The White House (2021b, May 26). *Statement by President Joe Biden on the Investigation into the Origins of COVID-19* [Statement]. www.whitehouse.gov/briefing-room/statements-releases/2021/05/26/statement-by-president-joe-biden-on-the-investigation-into-the-origins-of-covid-19/

The White House (2021c). *Statement by President Joseph Biden on the Investigation into the Origins of COVID-19* (May 26th). www.whitehouse.gov/briefing-room/statements-releases/2021/08/27/statement-by-president-joe-biden-on-the-investigation-into-the-origins-of-covid-%e2%81%a019/

United Nations Office for Disarmament Affairs (n.d.). *Secretary-General's Mechanism for Investigation of Alleged Use of Chemical and Biological Weapons (UNSGM).* https://disarmament.unoda.org/wmd/secretary-general-mechanism/

US Department of State (2021a, March 30). *Joint Statement on the WHO-Convened COVID-19 Origins Study* [Media Note]. www.state.gov/joint-statement-on-the-who-convened-covid-19-origins-study/

US Department of State (2021, January 15). *Activity at the Wuhan Institute of Virology* [Fact Sheet]. https://2017-2021.state.gov/fact-sheet-activity-at-the-wuhan-institute-of-virology/index.html

US Senate Committee on Health, Education, Labor and Pensions, Minority Oversight Staa (2022). *An Analysis of the Origins of the COVID-19 Pandemic. Interim Report*, October 2022.

Wade, N. (2021, May 5). The origin of COVID: Did people or nature open Pandora's box at Wuhan? *Bulletin of Atomic Scientists.* https://thebulletin.org/2021/05/the-origin-of-covid-did-people-or-nature-open-pandoras-box-at-wuhan/

World Health Organisation – China Joint Mission (2020, February 28). *Report of the WHO-China Joint Mission on Coronavirus Diseases 2019 (COVID-19)*. www.who. int/publications/i/item/report-of-the-who-china-joint-mission-on-coronavirus-disease-2019-(covid-19)

World Health Organisation (2020a, May 1). *Statement on the Third Meeting of the International Health Regulations (2005) Emergency Committee Regarding the Outbreak of coronavirus disease (COVID-19)* [Statement]. www.who.int/news/item/01-05-2020-statement-on-the-third-meeting-of-the-international-health-regulations-(2005)-emergency-committee-regarding-the-outbreak-of-coronavirus-disease-(covid-19)

World Health Organisation (2020b, November 6). *How WHO is Working to Track Down the Animal Reservoir of the SARS-CoV-2 virus.* www.who.int/news-room/feature-stories/detail/how-who-is-working-to-track-down-the-animal-reservoir-of-the-sars-cov-2-virus

World Health Organisation (2020c, January 23). *Statement on the First Meeting of the International Health Regulations (2005) Emergency Committee Regarding the Outbreak of Novel Coronavirus (2019-nCoV)* [Statement]. www.who.int/news/item/23-01-2020-statement-on-the-meeting-of-the-international-health-regulations-(2005)-emergency-committee-regarding-the-outbreak-of-novel-coronavirus-(2019-ncov)

World Health Organisation (2021a, February 11). *WHO Director-General's Opening Remarks at the Member States Briefing on COVID-19* [Opening Remarks]. www.who. int/director-general/speeches/detail/who-director-general-s-opening-remarks-at-the-member-states-briefing-on-covid-19---11-february-2021

World Health Organisation (2021b, February 9). *WHO Media Briefing from Wuhan on COVID-19 Mission* [Press Briefing]. www.who.int/multi-media/details/who-media-briefing-from-wuhan-on-covid-19-mission---9-february-2021

World Health Organisation (2021c, July 15). *COVID-19 Virtual Press Conference Transcript* [Press Briefing Transcript]. www.who.int/publications/m/item/covid-19-virtual-press-conference-transcript---15-july-2021

World Health Organisation (2021d, July 16). *WHO Director-General's Opening Remarks at the Member State Information Session on Origins* [Opening Statement]. www.who. int/director-general/speeches/detail/who-director-general-s-opening-remarks-at-the-member-state-information-session-on-origins

World Health Organisation (2021e, March 30). *WHO Director-General's Remarks at the Member State Briefing on the Report of the International Team Studying the Origins of SARS-CoV-2* [Director-General Remarks]. www.who.int/director-general/speeches/detail/who-director-general-s-remarks-at-the-member-state-briefing-on-the-report-of-the-international-team-studying-the-origins-of-sars-cov-2

World Health Organisation (2022, June 2). *Preliminary Report for the Scientific Advisory Group for the Origins of Novel Pathogens.* www.who.int/publications/m/item/scientific-advisory-group-on-the-origins-of-novel-pathogens-report

Wright, O. (2020, May 8). William Hague: Viruses are like weapons of mass destruction. *The Times.* www.thetimes.co.uk/article/william-hague-viruses-are-like-weapons-of-mass-destruction-h9nw2q50d

Zhen, S. H., Deverman, B. E., & Chan, Y. A. (2020). SARS-CoV-2 is well adapted for humans. What does this mean for re-emergence? *BioRxiv.* https://doi.org/10.1101/2020.05.01.073262

Zhou, P., Yang, X. L., Wang, X. G., Hu, B., Zhang, L., Zhang, W., Si, H. R., Zhu, Y., Li, B., Huang, H. D., Chen, H. D., Chen, J., Luo, Y., Guo, H., Jiang, R. D., Liu, M. Q., Chen, Y., Shen, X. R., Wang, X., Zheng, X. S., & Zhoa, K. (2020). A pneumonia outbreak associated with a new coronavirus of probable bat origin. *Nature*, 579, 270–273. https://doi.org/10.1038/s41586-020-2012-7

10 Conclusion

Patrick F. Walsh

Introduction

This chapter has three objectives. First, it will provide a final reflection on key themes arising from each chapter. There are many recurring themes across chapters and the first section will seek to combine many of these into larger 'meta-themes' to provide a foundation for anchoring further discussion in the final two sections of the chapter. The second section (Institutional and Policy Reform), informed by the previous thematic discussion will highlight areas where institutional and policy reform must take place across the health security intelligence enterprise in order to deliver more consistent, effective intelligence capabilities. Such reforms are essential if all stakeholders can harness their capabilities in ways that can better understand, prevent, mitigate and respond to future health security threats, risks and hazards. Thirdly, the chapter signposts a research agenda for researchers currently working across the health security intelligence spectrum as well as encouraging early career researchers to become more involved in this research in the future.

Key Themes Revisited

The first major theme identified early by Dahl (Chapter 2) is what role should national security intelligence agencies have in managing health security threats, risks and hazards? Should the prevention and response to health security related incidents and particularly emergencies such as COVID-19 be left solely up to public health authorities to manage? It would seem obvious that such agencies would play the major leading role in health security emergencies. Yet, as argued in this book, is there expertise and capabilities in the national security community that can support a whole of society strategy approach for the prevention and management of health security, threats, risks and hazards?

As stated several times throughout the book, COVID-19, beyond the significant public health impacts, also had profound economic, social and political ramifications – many of which are still being experienced globally. So, the implication of COVID-19 and some earlier health security threats, risks and hazards is that they can have wider (beyond public health) national security implications.

DOI: 10.4324/9781003335511-13

However, as discussed earlier, not all national security intelligence agencies played a role in dealing with COVID-19. Further, nor have they all necessarily in earlier decades been engaged actively in the management of other bio or health security threats and risks that have arisen including during the WMD in Iraq episode, Amerithrax and policy maker concerns over potentially growing bio-terrorism in the post-911 years. What national security intelligence agencies will be able to provide capabilities to assist in managing health security, threats, risks and hazards depends on several factors. These include: their mission identities, legislative powers, capabilities and the nature of the particular health security issue. COVID-19 has demonstrated also that some intelligence agencies have clearer mandates and missions that allow them to support and participate along with other non-national security stakeholders in managing health security issues. Though in a book that largely argues that national security intelligence agencies can and should play a greater role in managing health security threats, risks and hazards, we need to be mindful not all health security issues will have national security dimensions. And in these cases, their appropriate management is better managed exclusively by public health authorities or other scientific experts. However, as Walsh and Bernot suggest in Chapter 3 the inconsistency in the roles played by many national security intelligence agencies from 9/11 up to and including COVID-19 is not just a product of their actual mission identities and capabilities, but it is also in part due to long-standing inconsistent policy maker and institutional attention to health security, threats risks and hazards.

Chapter 3 showed that although there has definitely been political focus on bio and health threats, risks and hazards across some 'Five Eyes' countries since 9//11 (and even earlier), political rhetoric is not the same as profound, sustained and coordinated policy response that allows national security intelligence agencies to develop health security intelligence capabilities over time in ways that can adapt effectively as the threats, risk and hazard landscape changes. If policy makers and IC leaders are not sufficiently focusing on health security, threats, risks and hazards, or perhaps only during a crisis then it is difficult for national security intelligence agencies to determine what their mandates should be in these areas let alone building the right capabilities for any future role. This critical issue of what is the mandate and types of missions national security intelligence agencies should be involved in the health security context remains unresolved. It is critical that this fundamental issue is addressed by policy makers in the current post-COVID emergency period.

The second important theme again in Dahl's chapter is whether COVID-19 represents a historical intelligence failure? Dahl's chapter captures well the discordant voices on whether COVID-19 represents an intelligence failure. In some ways, a case can be made that it was perhaps in terms of the quality of intelligence provided, but also arguably more importantly was the warning provided to policy makers sufficiently impactful? Intelligence failures, as Betts reminds us, are often inevitable, complex and multifactorial. Insufficiencies at the collection and analytical stages can contribute to failure, but so too can broader IC organisational issues as well as decision-makers ignoring or not acting on the intelligence provided (Betts 1978). The theme of intelligence failure in the health security intelligence context will be returned to in the second section below (institutional and policy reform).

A third theme arising from Jennifer Hunt's Chapter 4 ('Disinformation: The COVID-19 Pandemic and Beyond') is, in the current post-acute COVID-19 period, what role should national security intelligence agencies play in monitoring disinformation propagated by state actors, religious/ideologically motivated terrorists and hosts of other issue-motivated groups that relate to health security issues? Malignant disinformation and misinformation relating to vaccines, public health interventions, trust in research, governments have only increased post-COVID not abated (Asiedu 2024; Gloor et al. 2024). Disinformation can be corrosive in liberal democracies causing further deterioration in government public health initiatives and the broader workings of democracy. We have seen how state actors such as China and Russia have taken advantage of disinformation campaigns during COVID-19, which suggests a clear mandate for national security intelligence agencies to better understand the nature of various state and non-state actors involved and the threat and risks they pose. Disinformation is both an issue that needs to be addressed at the policy and research levels and is discussed further below.

In Chapter 5, Gemma Bowsher provides several examples of how some 'Five Eyes' countries have taken further steps to improve how their intelligence communities might work more effectively on health security threats, risks and hazards in the post-emergency period of COVID-19. We have seen, for instance, on the issue of the origins of the pandemic how the US IC became involved, and it seems most 'Five Eyes' intelligence communities have been engaged in monitoring threat actors involved in disinformation. Through several examples, Bowsher provided a road map for developing more effective 'Five Eyes' intelligence capabilities post COVID-19. Chapter 5 underscores a fifth theme in the book, which is about the need for a more coherent strategic and operational approach by 'Five Eyes' intelligence communities to the management of health security threats, risks and hazards. We will come back to this theme in the next section (*Institutional and policy reform*).

In Chapter 6, Skillicorn discussed the clear technical challenges that remain in building better health security intelligence warning systems that can 'warn' or detect inherently rare health security or biological security events that may well have national security implications. His chapter frames in detail the many technical fundamentals that have led so far to sub-optimal warning systems both arguably used by public health authorities and ones that 'Five Eyes' intelligence communities may rely on to warn decision-makers about intentional and unintentional health security, threats, risks and hazards.

Skillicorn's chapter reminds us that there are no 'quick fixes' to improving health security intelligence warning and underscores a sixth theme that improving warning capabilities post-COVID 19 will remain difficult. Further, as noted in other chapters, more robust approaches will also require a significant investment in multi-disciplinary research to investigate both the technical and non-technical dimensions needed to optimise warning capabilities. This issue is discussed further in the remaining two sections.

In Chapter 7, Seumas Miller lists several large themes (biobank and database security, pandemics and dual use problems) where there remain significant moral problems that require policy-makers and 'Five Eyes' ICs engagement in order to manage more effectively biosecurity and broader health security threats, risks and hazards. Miller reminds us that while national security intelligence can serve a collective epistemic good, COVID-19 demonstrated several moral principles (privacy, confidentiality, autonomy rights, personal identity rights and ownership) are vulnerable to violation. And the ethical dilemmas raised in the collection and analysis of health security intelligence during the pandemic will need to be addressed more squarely by 'Five Eyes' ICs as they are confronted with post-COVID-19 biosecurity and health security, threats risks and hazards.

Kathleen Vogel in Chapter 8 ('Improving the Health Security Intelligence Workforce and Research Agenda') explored a range of critical issues relating to whether 'Five Eyes' intelligence communities currently are building a workforce capability that can play an effective role in managing health security and biological security threats, risks and hazards in a post-COVID 19 world. The second strand to Chapter 8 and related to building intelligence capability in this area, is how best to develop impactful research agendas that will also bring the cutting-edge knowledge and skills to build future capabilities. A central theme in Chapter 8 is therefore how to build future capability building within 'Five Eyes' intelligence communities in health security and biological security issues? Building on the excellent analysis by Vogel, this theme will be discussed further under the remaining two sections of the chapter.

Finally, Chapter 9 by Filippa Lentzos ('Managing Health Security Threats at the Multilateral Level') explored several critical themes around the role of multilateral institutions such the WHO, and other global countermeasures and compliance mechanisms aimed at preventing, disrupting and mitigating against emerging health security threats, risks and hazards beyond COVID-19. While highlighting the failures of the WHO multi-lateral efforts to investigate the origins of COVID-19, Lentzos argued persuasively that multilateral efforts to manage future health security threats, risks and hazards can be improved.

In particular, Lentzos' idea for development of an investigative body via WHO and its International Health Regulations to investigate ambiguous origin investigations in the future might gain traction in an increasingly fractured international community where security focused approaches such as an international treaty for future pandemic preparedness look increasingly unlikely. A key central theme emerging from this chapter is how best can 'Five Eyes' nations further bolster multilateral responses led by WHO and other international bodies to prevent, manage and investigate future health security threats, risks and hazards? What are the lessons that need to be learnt from failure points in WHO's investigation of COVID-19 origins and how can 'Five Eyes' nations and other like-minded liberal democracies encourage stronger and coordinated multilateral action on health security that promote robust global health responses, transparency and international confidence building?

Policy and Institutional Reform

Policy Reform

Reflecting on the themes discussed above, this section explores briefly what in an ideal world policy maker and 'Five Eyes' intelligence communities ought to do in order to better prepare for a post-COVID 19 health security environment – where a range of threats, risks and hazards may impact on the public health and broader national security interests of these nations and others globally.

'Five Eyes' countries are at risk of repeating earlier policy and institutional shortcomings seen in their responses to COVID-19 and previous health and biological security risks threats and hazards. At the time of writing, already four years after the acute phase of COVID-19 started, there is evidence that policy makers in some of these countries have set reforms in place to better respond to a future pandemic and perhaps other kinds of health security threats, risks or hazards. In the United States, under the Biden Administration, there have been several executive orders, strategies and policy documents (e.g., White House 2022a; White House 2022b; Biden 2022). In the UK the 2023 UK Biosecurity Strategy (2023) was launched (see Chapters 3 and 5 for further discussion). In the case of Canada at time of writing there has not been a substantive national government policy reform response to COVID-19 on the back of lessons learnt. However, in November 2023 a 643-page report by an independent national citizens inquiry was released into the appropriateness and efficacy of COVID-19 response by authorities there (NCI 2023). Time will tell whether policy initiatives in some of the above landmark initiatives across the 'Five Eyes' countries will be fully implemented and effective in preparing them for future health security events. However, despite these attempts at articulating policy reforms, four years after the COVID-19 pandemic started, it is likely that 'Five Eyes' policy makers have largely moved onto other more pressing national security issues nationally and internationally. Alongside policy-makers shifting attention away from health security threats, risks and pandemics, there are also national elections on the horizon in the US, and Canada, along with a recent change of government in the UK, which will distract further attention away from these issues. Given this attention shift by policy-makers away from health security issues in 'Five Eyes' capitals, it would not be surprising if their intelligence communities also reduce collection or analytical focus on health and biological security issues to what are considered more pressing collection and assessment priorities. In short, the crowded national security policy-agenda post-COVID-19, including Russia's invasion of Ukraine, China's coercive strategic and military posturing in the Indo-Pacific and instability in the Middle-East present dangerous threats and risks for 'Five Eyes' countries. Such complex and significant risks create an environment not necessarily conducive to their ICs reflecting deeply on what missions and mandates should national security intelligence agencies play in the health and biological threats, risks and hazards in the future?

Despite an inevitable shift in focus by policy-makers away from COVID-19 crisis management and responding to the pandemic's impact, there is still both the time and the need to make sure lessons can be learnt and captured from the whole of society response to the pandemic in order to provide a more comprehensive, robust and evidenced-based preparation for future health security, threats, risks and hazards. As noted above, in most 'Five Eyes' capitals governments in addition to announcing new policy strategies a number of independent (judicial) and/or parliamentary inquiries into various aspects of national responses to COVID-19 have been established. The key ones so far being, for example, the UK COVID-19 (Baroness Heather Hallett DBE) Inquiry announced in December 2022 (UK COVID-19 Inquiry nd), the Australian COVID-19 inquiry (led by Angela Jackson, Catherine Bennet and Robyn Kruk) announced in September 2023 (Chrysanthos 2023), and the New Zealand Royal Commission of Inquiry into New Zealand's COVID response announced in December 2022 (Ensor 2022). At time of writing all of three inquiries remain in progress. All three are independent judicial or expert-driven inquiries focused on COVID-19 issues such as preparedness, decision-making, role of government, data, legislation and a range of public health interventions. To date, there has been no independently commissioned inquiries into the US or Canadian government's response to COVID-19. In the US, and other 'Five Eyes' countries, there have been several parliamentary inquiries stood up during COVID-19. Some of these are continuing now into the post-emergency COVID-19 period. There are too many committees to name here, but examples are the US Senate Homeland Security and Governmental Affairs, the now concluded Australian Senate Select Committee on COVID-19 and in the UK multiple parliamentary committees such as the House of Commons Science and Technology Committee and the Health and Social Care and Science and Technology Committees have investigated a range of aspects regarding COVID-19 response and preparedness. While valuable insights are garnered from parliamentary/congressional committees the influence of partisan politics can and does constrain accounts of policy successes and failures as one or more political parties seeks to blame policy shortcomings on another party whilst its administration was in government during a particular stage of the COVID-19 pandemic.

It is also so far unclear based on the terms of reference and the records for these independent inquiries and parliamentary committees the extent to which they are fully capturing and evaluating the role of national security intelligence agencies in supporting whole of society responses to COVID-19 in 'Five Eyes' countries. Understandably, the focus of the various inquiries underway in the post-acute COVID-19 period have a public health and social impact emphasis. While this is appropriate, inquiry results may be insufficient if they do not investigate what activities non-public health stakeholders such as national security intelligence agencies were involved in to support government's COVID-19 response, whether they were sufficient and effective and how this knowledge might inform the roles 'Five Eyes' intelligence communities should take on now in order to prepare for future health security, threats, risks and hazards.

It is currently unknown the extent to which 'Five Eyes' intelligence communities have undertaken any internal reviews of their support to COVID-19 including identifying challenges and capability gaps to more effectively support whole of society responses to future health security threats, risks and hazards. But as noted in previous chapters – in the US, most starkly, but also in other 'Five Eyes' countries – aspects of governments and their bureaucratic handling of COVID-19 has become politicised (see Chapter 3) This raises the questions about whether both the current independent and various parliamentary inquiries can provide both non-partisan and comprehensive oversight of the role of IC agencies played in managing aspects of COVID-19 and the extent to which they are preparing for any future health security, threats risks? Are there other feasible review options that can provide oversight of the role of 'Five Eyes' ICs during COVID-19 and their mandates into the future? In the case of Australia, the government has commissioned two former senior intelligence and policy leaders Richard Maud and Heather Smith to review the state of the national intelligence community (NIC). These independent reviews are done regularly in Australia (every five to seven years). The last in 2017 ushered in significant changes to Australia's intelligence community including the establishment of the Office of National Intelligence and the expansion of the NIC to ten agencies (Walsh 2021; and L'Estrange and Merchant 2017). The terms of reference for the current 2024 independent intelligence review did not include any government request for the reviewers to examine how the NIC responded to COVID-19 (Independent Intelligence Review 2023). However, Walsh and Bernot (see Chapter 3) provided in their written submission to their reviewers areas (including but not limited to governance, early warning and workforce) where they should investigate regarding the NIC's response to COVID (Walsh and Bernot 2023; Walsh et al. 2023). The reviewer's report is due to be released later in 2024 and at this point it is unclear whether reporting on how the NIC engaged with national COVID-19 response will be included in their report. But it does provide at least for one 'Five Eyes' nation another independent non-partisan opportunity to review NIC capabilities relating to COVID-19 and potentially how they may be configured to manage future health security, threats, risks and hazards.

Leaving aside what might be included in the next Australian independent intelligence review, concerns over the remit of current independent inquiries and the extent to which existing of future parliamentary reviews have become politicised, it is argued here that in each 'Five Eyes' country it will still (after four years) be beneficial for an independent non-partisan review into how the national security intelligence agencies participated in supporting COVID-19 responses. An independent non-partisan review should include an investigation into their effectiveness and how they might position their capabilities to meet emerging health security threats, risks and hazards. Several scholars and commentators have suggested for several years now that governments need the equivalent of a '9/11 Commission' independent non-partisan inquiry into national COVID-19 responses (Chyba et al. 2021; Gronvall 2020). Regardless of opinion on the outcomes of the 9/11 Commission, the two-year review resulted in a detailed report, which included many ideas about how the US IC might reconfigure its capabilities to deal with counter-terrorism in the future. However, the political will – arguably in all 'Five Eyes' countries – for such a detailed forensic (9/11 Commission equivalent) review of national security intelligence capabilities used during COVID-19 in extended public hearings has likely gone. Nonetheless, it is still possible and desirable for 'Five Eyes' governments to commission more scaled-down, independent non-partisan inquiries into how their respective intelligence communities engaged in COVID-19 and the lessons to be learnt. Much like the regular Australian independent intelligence reviews, independent expert reviewers can be appointed, and they can interview all key players and produce both a classified and unclassified report that serves both policy maker requirements and promotes public accountability into the actions of their intelligence communities during the pandemic.

There are several areas that reviewers should focus on, all of which are central themes identified in this book by contributors. Due to space limitations these will not be repeated here. However, critical areas ripe for review are governance, which includes what mandates and missions each IC agency should play in health security threats, risks and hazards? What agency should lead the coordination of the whole of IC response and how should mission deconfliction take place? Another governance issue is how should ICs work with public health, biotechnology, private sector and other stakeholders in carrying out this mission in the future? Other critical review topics include to what extent COVID-19 was an intelligence failure and if is it possible to build better warning capabilities for future similar health security threats, risks and hazards. Other important review themes could investigate how best to lever external expertise yet also building better internal subject matter expertise within the ICs workforce? While researchers should remain realistic about the prospects that policy makers may not invest in these much-needed independent health security intelligence reviews, the downside of not doing so leaves 'Five Eyes' intelligence communities reverting to patchwork reforms as each agency moves on to other more pressing business. And any IC reforms that do occur are at risk of being done in siloes rather than a whole of IC approach to reform which unfortunately has been the fallback position to several reform efforts pre-COVID-19.

National Health or Biological Security Strategies

The second important strand to improving policy and institutional reform in responding to health security threats, risks and hazards in the future is the need for each 'Five Eyes' to develop national health or biological security strategies. This is not to suggest that no strategic work has been completed by policy makers on how to respond to 'future COVID-19s'. Previous chapters, particularly Chapters 3 and 5, have given several examples of policies and strategic initiatives some 'Five Eyes' capitals have implemented during and after COVID-19. For example, in Chapter 5 Bowsher discussed the revised 2023 UK Biosecurity Strategy, which clarifies roles and taskings and outlines how workflows and relationships between intelligence functions such as those within the Cabinet Office, the Ministry of Defence (MOD), and other security-oriented functions are mapped in relation to the UK Health Security Agency (UKHSA), Foreign Commonwealth and Development Office (FCDO) and other government departments (HM Gov 2023). The reader is referred back to Chapters 3 and 5 for granular discussion of more recent policy and strategic initiatives in response to COVID-19. But leaving aside the existence of these initiatives, it is uncertain whether this planning sufficiently provides a clear roadmap for all stakeholders (national security intelligence agencies included) to identify and operationalise their mandates, missions and capabilities to prevent, disrupt, mitigate and respond to future health security issues. In an idea world, a best practice public policy response here would be informed by all the inquiries currently underway as mentioned earlier, as well as the independent health security intelligence reviews advocated for in the last section. Though recognising it is not always possible for strategies to be informed by other parallel processes, it is now important for governments to release *national health or biological security strategies* that provide sufficiently detailed framework for a 'whole of society' response to health and biological security issues over the next several (five to seven) years. Such a strategy should be sufficiently detailed yet remain high level. A good template to develop these may be national cyber-security strategies across 'Five Eyes' countries. National cyber-security strategies are instructive because they generally articulate a comprehensive role for all critical stakeholders including how the public also has a role in protecting themselves from cyber threats. It's this 'whole of society' approach that seems to be still lacking in current policy and strategic initiatives on health and biological security.

A national health security strategy will clearly contain different content in each 'Five Eyes' country depending on the country's political institutions, size of research and biotechnology communities, legislation, governance and oversight mechanisms. But regardless of distinct national characteristics, such strategies should include similar broad components. Here, I am suggesting six components. The first component should describe the current and emerging health/biological security landscape. In other words what are the threats, risks and hazards and how are they evolving? The second component needs to outline comprehensively the role of key stakeholders who to varying degrees will need to engage with the strategy. These include, but are not limited to: public health, animal health, IC agencies, the research and biotechnology sectors and the public. For each listing of a stakeholder there needs to be an articulation of the relevant governance arrangements and how common missions are identified, integrated and deconflicted. A third component should address health and biological security critical infrastructure. This section may include the role and responsibilities of various stakeholders (national security agencies, public health, multi-lateral institutions, regulation, and the biotechnology and research sectors). COVID-19 demonstrated how supply chains in medical supplies (e.g. vaccines, ventilators, and personal protective equipment) and how pandemic lockdowns also impacted adversely on the broader supply of other goods and services across 'Five Eyes' economies. A fourth component in a strategy could provide a strategic framework for building national capabilities. This section could usefully include how a nation grows its national health security workforce not just in national security agencies, but supporting the growth of a security workforce in the pharmaceutical, health, biotechnology research and innovation industries that in the future will have leadership and managerial responsibility for countering potential health security, threats, risks and hazard particularly in the private and public sector. A fifth component could focus on regional and international measures that a nation could seek to influence that fosters confidence-building measures, norms and standards for addressing emerging health security, threats, risks and hazards. A final section in the strategy would map out the evaluation metrics governments and stakeholders would be held accountable for delivering at various phases or milestones of the strategy. A national health or biological security strategy of course is insufficient on its own to push policy and institution reform in health or biological security post-COVID. Each critical stakeholder, including national security intelligence agencies would need to develop in collaboration with national governments their action plans to provide an operational response to the strategy.

In the action plans of each 'Five Eyes' intelligence community, a granular discussion of topics identified in the higher-level strategy would be expected. Action plans should lay out a framework that explains clearly how each 'Five Eyes' intelligence community and each agency within these communities, would operationalise mandates, functions, governance and oversight activities. It's likely that there would be some overlap between several activities in an action plan. For example, under a 'prevention' heading further description of activities may include: early warning systems, managing disinformation, security vetting, establishing intelligence collection and assessment priorities. Under 'mitigation' and 'response' headings, many of the activities listed under 'prevention' might remain relevant but will have a different operational focus. Added to a 'mitigation' or 'response' phase of an action plan may be intelligence-led disruption activities, attribution investigations, counter-intelligence/deception detection by state actors, critical infrastructure protection, compliance and logistical support by national security intelligence agencies in broader public health activities – such as public health orders, and contact tracing where appropriate legally and with due consideration to ethical issues (see Chapter 6, Miller). Much of the policy and institutional reforms suggested here can also be informed by identifying lessons learnt but assessing what is good practice also requires an investment by ICs in research projects that identify ways capabilities and processes can be improved. We turn now to a final reflection on research priorities.

Research Agenda

In Chapter 8, Kathleen Vogel presented six research priorities areas related to health security intelligence relevant for 'Five Eyes' ICs. These are: climate change, emerging bio-sciences and technology, bio-data/algorithmic security risks, disinformation/misinformation, resolving health security disputes amongst experts and early warning systems. Many of these research priority areas have also been identified thematically in other chapters in the book. Additionally some of the research priorities and challenges are already openly recognised by IC agencies (e.g., early warning, disinformation/misinformation and resolving disputes among health security experts). However, less is known about the IC's interest or investment in other research priorities identified.

This section provides a final reflection on some of the research priorities identified by Vogel and other contributors in the book. It explores what additional considerations need to be taken into account in approaching the design, funding, coordination and management of research priorities of relevance to 'Five Eyes' IC agencies. The purpose is not to provide granular or prescriptive projects for research areas explored. Rather it is to argue for both a sustained and multi-disciplinary investment in research within and across 'Five Eyes' ICs to address the current capability gaps each research priority area represents. Given limited space, I will focus only on three research priorities identified on Vogel's list: emerging bio-sciences and technology, early warning and disinformation/misinformation. These three have been selected because of how frequently they were discussed in previous chapters, in the literature and with discussions with IC practitioners. In short, a strong case can be made for them being priority investment research areas by 'Five Eyes' ICs.

In terms of the first research priority – emerging bio-sciences and technology there are a range of critical unknowns and knowledge gaps across 'Five Eyes' ICs about how the rapid acceleration of innovations in synthetic biology and bio-technology may create security dilemmas (Walsh 2018; Vogel and Ouargraham-Gormley 2018; Watters et al. 2021; West and Gronvall 2020; Paris 2023). Firstly, it would be erroneous to suggest that 'Five Eyes' ICs are not currently sponsoring research to better understand the security implications of synthetic biology and biotechnology. The literature suggests some ICs are particularly focused on funding research projects in synthetic biology that seek to improve intelligence capabilities and enable more effective responses to broader bio-defence missions (Walsh 2018; Trump et al. 2021). Similarly, the literature shows that ICs continue to sponsor research and consultancy expertise on issues such as the attribution of both natural and various synthetic bio-agents in order to ascertain whether they might be synthesised deceptively for malevolent intentions such as bioterrorism (Worobey et al. 2022; Callisher et al. 2021; Walsh et al. 2023). One area of synthetic biology and biotechnology where ICs are showing increasing concern for several years now is genomic editing. In February 2016, Director of National Intelligence James R. Clapper issued a warning in the ODNI's annual *World Wide Threat Assessment of the United States Intelligence Community* that genomic editing could be misused deliberately or unintentionally to create harmful biological agents or products (Clapper 2016). While the announcement by the then US Director of National Intelligence highlighted an interest in genomic editing, it also arguably demonstrated how little most 'Five Eyes' IC understood about the potential national security implications of these increasingly used techniques (e.g. CRISPR) by the broader scientific and biotechnology industries. Eight years on from the 2016 DNI announcement, there is likely an increased understanding of the national security dimensions of genomic editing like CRISPR within some 'Five Eyes' IC agencies. Nonetheless, I would argue both the collection and assessment capabilities on the potential misuse, threats and risks associated with genomic editing are not optimal. In short, better intelligence collection and analysis of threats, risks and hazards posed by the intentional weaponization of synthetic biology and biotechnology techniques and technologies (like CRISPR) can only be achieved by more sustained investment by IC agencies to gain evidenced based multi-disciplinary knowledge that can better assess associated threats, risks and hazards. This statement is obvious. But what is less certain is the extent to which post-COVID 'Five Eyes' IC agencies that have a mandate to collect and assess against health and biological security threats, risks and hazards are committed longer term to obtaining this evidence-based multi-disciplinary-based knowledge. Are the almost exponential innovations in synthetic biology and biotechnology that CRISPR represents viewed by many in the IC as being too complex and likely at best low probability/high impact threats/risks? Does the potentially overwhelming complexity of genomic editing almost as default relegate them to low collection and assessment priorities by ICs? It's true that already over-stretched ICs do not have the bandwidth nor need to chase every imagined security implication of all the innovations in synthetic biology and biotechnology. But given the critical centrality CRISPR and other genomic editing techniques and technologies currently have and likely will continue to have in the global biotechnology sector, ICs do need to develop more granular evidenced-based collection and analysis of their security implications.

The recent COVID pandemic only highlights starkly the importance by ICs to better understand the security implications associated with genomic editing. As noted earlier, the scientific and medical response to COVID-19 underscored how innovations such as genomic editing became the backbone of developing rapid detection tests for SAR-CoV-2 and are expected to play an increasing role in the development of mRNA vaccines for COVID and other viral diseases in the future. The rapidity in which mRNA vaccines produced by companies like Pfizer and Moderna was possible in large part because of the growing automation of pharmaceutical bio-processing – itself facilitated by the integration of cyber/AI enabled and bioprocessing, which in turn allowed the faster design, manufacturing and delivery of research outputs such as vaccines.

However, attacks against global pharmaceuticals during COVID-19 underscored several vulnerabilities in critical health infrastructure and supply chains. Further, as discussed earlier, the malicious cyber-hacking of big pharmaceuticals such as Pfizer BioNTech to steal IP related to mRNA vaccines during COVID-19 can impact on the political, health, economic and social wellbeing of countries (Walsh 2022, 335–355). Additionally, such state-sponsored and non-state actor attacks on biotechnology industries can impact scientific collaboration. A reduced willingness by countries to share scientific data could, in turn, result potentially in delays in scientific discoveries that harm the health of patients (Walsh 2022, 335–355). In short, these recent examples from the acute COVID-19 period demonstrate that 'Five Eyes' ICs do have cause for concern that state and non-state actors *may* maliciously exploit both the public and private synthetic biology and biotechnology sectors. It also means that as the use of genomic technologies and techniques become increasingly ubiquitous in these sectors they *could* be exploited by malevolent individual, state and non-state actors for ideological, political, strategic and economic ends.

The significant knowledge gap within 'Five Eyes' ICs about how genomic editing techniques and technologies could be misused by malevolent actors and what risks these would pose cannot be met solely within ICs. Although some genomic editing techniques are becoming scientifically more accessible and easier to use, there are as Paris suggests a range of barriers (technical, social, operational, logistical and ethical) that for the most part still need to be overcome even by skilled scientists, who may be working for state and non-state actors to weaponize these techniques (Paris 2023, 213). There is even lesser probability that a threat actor with lower laboratory skills, knowledge and experience could 'weaponise' CRISPR to create a bio-weapon (ibid.). Nonetheless, the complexities and nuances about *what threat actors* and *how CRISPR* could be weaponised needs a deeper, longer-term multi-disciplinary research investment by 'Five Eyes' ICs than hitherto has been the case. 'Five Eyes' IC capability funding needs to harness a collaboration of molecular biologists, AI, biotechnology, intelligence studies, psychology, regulatory/legal and ethical scholars to ensure there are overtime comprehensive improvements in what genomic technologies and techniques are likely to be misused by bad actors and how these threats, risks and hazards are best mitigated against – while not blocking progress in legitimate application of genomic editing in the synthetic biology and biotechnology sectors (Nester 2022; Paris 2022; Valdivia-Granda 2019; Vogel & Ouagrham-Gormley 2018; Wang et al. 2023; Watters et al. 2021; West and Gronvall 2020).

The second research priority area that also needs sustained investment by all 'Five Eyes' ICs is health security intelligence early warning systems. Several chapters focused on the technical, policy challenges and deficiencies associated with the failure of health security intelligence early warning systems used by public health and national security agencies leading up to and including COVID-19 (see Chapters 2, 3 and 6). Similar to genomic editing, again it is not that 'Five Eyes' ICs are not aware of the need to develop more robust health security intelligence early warning systems, but being aware is one thing and investing in research and development to improve these systems is another matter. During COVID-19 and now in the current acute pandemic period an increasing number of researchers are working on various aspects of how to improve early warning systems (Gu and Li 2020; Mehta et al. 2020; Newell 2021; MacIntyre et al. 2023; Coocia 2023; Han and Ginsberg 2019). Governments rhetoric, as noted in the above section post-COVID-19, has also declared nationals and the international community needs to develop better early warning systems. For example, work underway at the national level US CDC Centre for Forecasting and Outbreak and Analytics, signals scope to enhance existing epidemiological intelligence with lessons from national security early warning principles (see Chapter 5). The newly established (January 2024) Australia's Centre for Disease Control at this point also looks like it might develop over time an horizon-scanning early warning capability in the future (Australian Centre for Disease Control n.d). Similarly at the international and multilateral level the WHO with assistance from member states has established the WHO Hub for Pandemic and Epidemic Intelligence (WHO 2021). And as Bowsher argued in Chapter 5, for some in the WHO there has been more focus on intelligence (national security) based approaches to improve traditional epidemiological data to monitor disease and control measures on a real-time basis.

Yet the literature shows a diverse field of disciplines currently engaged in 'early warning' against pandemics. Some appear to be just trying to automate already existing traditional disease surveillance systems, others seek to improve on longstanding digital epidemiologic surveillance systems – while others seek to develop early warning that may detect indicators of emerging novel diseases that may have pandemic potential. Hence, the research on early warning can be both diverse and confusing as it stretches across diverse temporal contexts. Confusing because different researchers and practitioners have different views on what 'early warning means' in their contexts. On one end of the spectrum, there are early warning systems to allow traditional contact tracers heads up where an already significant disease outbreak may be heading next and on the other, systems exist that attempt to provide longer-term strategic warning of indicators that novel disease of pandemic potential is on the horizon. The early warning literature can also be siloed within or across only a few disciplines such as machine learning and AI aspects (MacIntyre et al. 2023), while others focus more on epidemiological warnings for public health contact tracing and predicting and modelling disease spread (Donelle et al. 2023). What the bulk of this literature shows is the broader early warning systems that have existed now for several decades have produced patchy results as shown in their application against the initial onslaught of the COVID-19 pandemic (Parker et al. 2022; Simek et al. 2018; Sweeney 2020; Syrowatka et al. 2021; Donelle et al. 2023; Wilson 2017). As Skillicorn (see Chapter 6) reminds us health security intelligence warning systems are 'not, at present, so sophisticated'. 'While most countries have some form of disease early-warning system, the COVID-19 pandemic showed that these are often too sluggish to respond to exponentially increasing cases, and struggle with multiple, incoherent sources of data' (Chapter 6).

Skillicorn explored some areas of data analytics such as linear configuration and non-linear configuration spaces in addition to Bayesian approaches that may help with anomaly detection and improve functionality which is critical for building early warning systems for unknown novel diseases of pandemic potential. However, as noted in Chapter 6, many of these developments in data analytics require active research to further assess their utility to building better health security intelligence warning systems that could provide longer strategic warning than has been the case with systems so far.

The inconsistent performance of so many early warning systems before and leading up to COVID-19 requires a significant investment in research and development of better health security intelligence warning systems that obviously lead to better public health outcomes. But also warning systems should also have utility for 'Five Eyes' ICs where novel or even 'suspicious' disease outbreaks may require their involvement in understanding them as early as possible in order to warn policy makers of any potential national security dimensions of outbreaks.

What COVID-19 highlighted was a proliferation of digital technologies used by WHO, nations, their public health agencies (local, regional and national levels), and the private sector. Hardware such as CCTV, drones and digital thermometers were all used. In terms of software, aggregate mobile data, data from private companies, Apple- Google API, crowdsourcing technology and immigration databases were also exploited. Finally, in respect to technology, health insurance date bases, google trends data, geofencing, mobile phones apps, QR codes, social media and remote monitoring were all used (Donelle et al. 2023, 7–8).

With so many public and private stakeholders now trying to develop more effective early warning systems post-COVID-19, there are significant knowledge and capability challenges for 'Five Eyes' ICs on what kind of health security intelligence warning systems would best support their mandates in managing emerging health and biological threats, risks and hazards.

Skillicorn and the broader literature demonstrate the significant technical challenges in building better building better health security intelligence warning systems that can 'warn' or detect inherently rare events. While there is historical and, in some parts, deep expertise on early warning capabilities within some 'Five Eyes' ICs, the application of existing principles and capabilities do not necessarily translate into detecting emerging complex health and biological security issues. Now is the opportunity for the 'Five Eyes' ICs to engage in deep collaboration with trusted researchers to unravel the challenges in progressing more reliable health security intelligence early warning systems. Again, along with all the research challenges discussed in this chapter and the book 'Five Eyes' ICs need to invest for the longer term in multi-disciplinary research collaborations that will identify the range of technical and non-technical issues currently constraining better early warning systems in this area. Much has already been said about some of the current technical (data analytics /machine learning) barriers constrain the development of more responses health security intelligence early warning systems. But from a range of multi-disciplinary perspectives there are many other challenges that will not be solved if early warning systems become captured solely by public health or machine learning experts – however essential they are in providing part of the solution. Other, perhaps even more fundamental, questions need to be explored. For example, what kind of early warning system do 'Five Eyes' ICs need? What levels of decision-making should it be focused on: tactical, operational or strategic – or a combination of all three? What kind of indicators are most valid to include and what public and private data should be collected to inform those indicators (e.g. hospital visits, social media, genomic surveillance data, contact tracing)? Additionally, as Miller noted in Chapter 7, what non-national security intelligence information such as public health data should be shared with 'Five Eyes' ICs for this warning purpose? What internal governance processes within 'Five Eyes' ICs need to be resolved in order for intelligence analysts and relevant leadership chains to assess the validity and reliability of warning triggers coming from various different IC agencies?

The final and third research challenge, which also has urgency, is for 'Five Eyes' ICs to sponsor multi-disciplinary research collaborations on how to best manage disinformation and misinformation propagated by threat actors that can, as we saw during COVID-19, impact on trust in governments, their public health interventions, scientists and the resilience of democracies in general. As pointed out by Jennifer Hunt (Chapter 4), the impact of COVID-19 disinformation continues at a pace even though the acute pandemic stage looks to be over. State, non-state and conspiracy theory driven individuals continue to fuel narratives about the perceived danger of vaccines, public health expertise and mistrust in the government particularly in the United States. While progress is being made by some ICs to better understand disinformation in general – particularly as it may involve foreign state actor interference, a greater, more sophisticated understanding of threat and risk taxonomies as they relate to health and biological security issues is critical. Being able to classify threat and risk is critical if liberal democracies are to better prepare for any future substantial health security event. It is particularly important in supporting government's communication of valid public health messaging while detecting and constraining the physical and virtual malignant messaging by threat actors who seek to ignite social disharmony and violence. Again, as with the other two research priorities, the production of better-quality knowledge and evidence that 'Five Eyes' ICs can use to play their role in managing disinformation requires a multi-disciplinary research design. A collaborative approach that includes researchers in psychology, political science, communication studies, AI, regulation, law, ethics, public health and national security amongst others can all usefully bring something to the table. Part of this research obviously needs to focus not just on the quicker detection and classification of threat actors, but provide ICs with support in deciding what role they should play in designing counter health security-related disinformation narratives. In particular, to what extent and circumstances where trust in ICs across liberal democracies is low should they be seen to curate, disrupt or deliver counter-narrative interventions? And to what extent could other non-intelligence public sector agencies or the private sector take this up? Arguably, many of these questions remain unresolved.

The Future

Finally, to circle back to the three aims listed in Chapter 1. The book seeks to contribute to ongoing debates about health and biological security and its national security implications post-COVID-19 (Frutos et al. 2020). First, it investigated what roles 'Five Eyes' intelligence communities played (along with other key stakeholders such as public health agencies) in managing COVID-19. Second, it assessed the challenges and lessons learnt for 'Five Eyes' intelligence communities in how they have engaged in managing aspects of the COVID-19 pandemic. Third, how may 'Five Eyes' intelligence communities play more effective roles in managing future health security threats and risks – whether these are intentional (bioterrorism and bio crimes), accidental (accidental laboratory releases) or unintentional (pandemics) in origin.

There is still much to learn from how democracies such as 'Five Eyes' countries responded to COVID-19 and what this means for designing better whole of society resilience against future significant health and biological security events. In any current and future public policy reforms post COVID-19, we argue a truly effective 'whole of society' resilience to emerging health security threats, risks and hazards must also include articulating a clearer mandate and enhanced capabilities of 'Five Eyes' ICs in order to play their part in them. However, what is not understood sufficiently is what role both, strategically and operationally, intelligence communities should play in a world that presents a range of potential yet complex health security threats, risks and hazards? The book also sought to begin unravelling other key questions. These include: what unique value can the 'Five Eyes' intelligence communities offer to public health authorities and other responders as part of an all-hazards approach to managing such threats, risks and hazards? What are the boundaries between what resources and capabilities our intelligence agencies can bring to bear in managing health security threats and risks; and what is the role of other public and private stakeholders?

This book fills a gap in the intelligence studies literature about what role 'Five Eyes' intelligence enterprises should play in supporting policy makers, researchers, the public and private health sector, in understanding health security threats/risks in a post-COVID-19 world.

The edited collection also brought together a multi-disciplinary approach to understanding emerging health security threats and hazards. In particular, the volume is a fusion of perspectives from experts with extensive backgrounds in national security intelligence, and other fields including but not limited to biodefence, public health, ethics, computer science, medicine, biotechnology, and science and technology – to better understand emerging health security threats/ risks/hazards and to determine the role national security intelligence could play in managing them.

There is no pretence that this edited volume comprehensively assesses the roles played by all 'Five Eyes' intelligence agencies during COVID-19. Some countries have received wider coverage than others mostly due to a greater availability of open-source information and where contributors are from. COVID-19 remains for many countries a sensitive political issue and details about what ICs did or didn't do during this period is likewise sensitive – hence the calls in the book for an independent inquiry in each country. The book has its limitations both from disciplinary and scope perspectives. The approach has been deliberately multi-disciplinary, but the analysis would have been richer with additional voices from a range of other fields such as epidemiology, animal health, disease ecology and relevant stakeholders in the private sector. It is hoped nonetheless that the collection will generate broader and deeper discussions from researchers, ICs, policy makers, public health, biotechnology about the national security implications of health and biological security threats, risks and hazards post-COVID-19. It is hoped that the book will encourage more policy and research activity around the issues presented and provide a foundation where the many gaps in health and biological security knowledge over time will be filled.

References

Asiedu, K. (2024, 15 March). *Four Years After Shelter in Place, COVID-19 Misinformation Persists*. Politifact. The Poynter Institute. www.politifact.com/article/2024/mar/15/four-years-after-shelter-in-place-covid-19-misinfo/

Betts, R. K. (1978). Analysis, War, and Decision: Why Intelligence Failures Are Inevitable. *World Politics*, 31(1), 61–89. doi:10.2307/2009967

Biden, J. R. (2022). Biden-Harris White House National Security Strategy, October 2022. Collections, 2022, 10–12.

Calisher, C., et al. (2021). Science Not Speculation is Essential to Determine how SARS-COV-2 Reached Humans. *Lancet*, 1–3, Published Online July 5, 2021. doi:10.1016/S0140-6736(21)01419-7

Cho, A. (2020). Artificial Intelligence Systems Aim to Sniff Out Signs of COVID 19 Outbreaks. *Science*, 368, 810–811. doi:10.1126/science.368.6493.810

Chrysanthos, N. (2023, 6 November). What's the Evidence? Inquiry to Probe Rationale for COVID Lockdowns. *Sydney Morning Herald*. www.smh.com.au/politics/federal/evidence-trail-inquiry-to-probe-path-to-covid-lockdowns-20231106-p5ehxi.html

Chyba, C. F., Cassel, C. K., Graham, S. L., Holdren, J. P., Penhoet, E., Press, W. H., & Varmus, H. (2021). Create a COVID-19 Commission. *Science*, 374(6570), 932–935. doi:10.1126/science.abk0029

Clapper, J. (2016). *Statement for the Record*. Worldwide Threat Assessment of the US Intelligence Community. Armed Services Committee, US Congress.

Dahl, E. J. (2023). *The COVID-19 Intelligence Failure: Why Warning Was Not Enough*. Washington, DC: Georgetown University Press.

Donelle, L., Comer, L., Hiebert, B., Hall, J., Shelley, J. J., Smith, M. J., ... & Facca, D. (2023). Use of Digital Technologies for Public Health Surveillance During the COVID-19 Pandemic: A Scoping Review. *Digital Health*, 9, 20552076231173220.

Ensor, J. (2022). Royal Commission of Inquiry into New Zealand's COVID Response Announced News Hub, 5 December. www.newshub.co.nz/home/politics/2022/12/royal-commission-of-inquiry-into-new-zealand-s-covid-19-response-announced.html

Frutos, R., Lopez Roig, M., Serra-Cobo, J., & Devaux, C. A. (2020). COVID-19: The Conjunction of Events Leading to the Coronavirus Pandemic and Lessons to Learn for Future Threats. *Frontiers in Medicine*, 7(223). doi:10.3389/fmed.2020.00223

Gloor, P. A., Grippa, F., Fronzetti Colladon, A., Przegalinska, A., Oet, M., Zhou, X., & Takko, T. (2024). *Handbook of Social Computing*. Edward Elgar Publishing.

Gronvall, G. K. (2020). The Scientific Response to COVID-19 and Lessons for Security. *Survival*, 62(3), 77–92. https://doi.org/10.1080/00396338.2020.1763613

Gu, E. & Li, L. (2020). Crippled Community Governance and Suppressed Scientific/Professional Communities: A Critical Assessment of Failed Early Warning for the COVID-19 Outbreak in China. *Journal of Chinese Governance*, 5(2), 160–177. doi:10.1080/23812346.2020.1740468

Han, B. & Ginsberg, J. (2019, October 3). *Using AI to Predict and Pre-empt Epidemics*. New York: Cary Institute of Ecosystem Studies. www.caryinstitute.org/news-insights/lecture-video/using-ai-predict-preempt-epidemics

HMG (2023). *UK Biological Security Strategy*. London.

Independent Intelligence Review (2023). Terms of Reference. Department of Prime Minister and Cabinet, Canberra. www.pmc.gov.au/resources/2024-independent-intelligence-review-terms-reference

L'Estrange, M. & Merchant, S. (2017). *2017 Independent Intelligence Review*. Canberra: Commonwealth of Australia.

MacIntyre, C. R., Chen, X., Kunasekaran, M., Quigley, A., Lim, S., Stone, H., Paik, H.-Y., et al. (2023). Artificial Intelligence in Public Health: The Potential of Epidemic Early Warning Systems. *Journal of International Medical Research*, 51(3), 03000605231159335.

Mehta, M. C., Katz, I. T., & Jha, A. K. (2020). Transforming Global Health with AI. *New England Journal of Medicine, 382*(9), 791–793. doi:10.1056/NEJMp1912079

NCI (2023). Inquiry into the Appropriateness and Efficacy of the COVID-19 Response in Canada. https://nationalcitizensinquiry.b-cdn.net/wp-content/uploads/2023/12/FINAL-REPORT-Volume-1-2-3-Inquiry-into-the-Appropriateness-and-Efficacy-of-the-COVID-19-Response-in-Canada-December-21-2023.pdf

Nestor, M. W. & Wilson, R. L. (2022). *Anticipatory Ethics and the Use of CRISPR in Humans.* Cham, Switzerland: Springer.

Newell, B. (2021). Introduction: Surveillance and the COVID-19 Pandemic: Views from Around the World. *Surveillance & Society, 19*(1), 81–84.

Paris, K. (2022). *Genome Editing and Biological Weapons: Assessing the Risk of Misuse.* Cham: Springer International Publishing AG.

Parker, C. F. & Stern, E. K. (2022). The Trump Administration and the COVID-19 Crisis: Exploring the Warning-Response Problems and Missed Opportunities of a Public Health Emergency. *Public Administration, 100*(3), 616–632. https://doi.org/10.1111/padm.12843

Simek, O., et al. (2018). XLab: Early Indications and Warnings from Open Source Data with Application to Biological Threat. Paper presented at the Proceedings of the 51st Hawaii International Conference on System Sciences, University of Hawaii.

Sweeney, Y. (2020). Tracking the Debate on COVID-19 Surveillance Tools. *Nature Machine Intelligence, 2*(6), 301–304. doi:10.1038/s42256-020-0194-1

Syrowatka, A., Kuznetsova, M., Alsubai, A., Beckman, A. L., Bain, P. A., Craig, K. J. T., & Bates, D. W. (2021). Leveraging Artificial Intelligence for Pandemic Preparedness and Response: A Scoping Review to Identify Key Use Cases. *npj Digital Medicine, 4*(1), 96. doi:10.1038/s41746-021-00459-8

Trump, B. D., Florin, M.-V., Perkins, E., & Linkov, I. (2021). *Emerging Threats of Synthetic Biology and Biotechnology: Addressing Security and Resilience Issues.* Dordrecht, Netherlands, The Springer Netherlands.

UK COVID-19 Inquiry (n.d.). UK COVID-19 Inquiry. https://covid19.public-inquiry.uk/about/

Valdivia-Granda, W. A. (2019). Big Data and Artificial Intelligence for Biodefense: A Genomic-Based Approach for Averting Technological Surprise. In *Defense Against Biological Attacks* (pp. 317–327). Springer.

Vogel, K. M. & Ouagrham-Gormley, S. B. (2018). Anticipating Emerging Biotechnology Threats: A Case Study of CRISPR. *Politics and the Life Sciences, 37*(2), 203–219. doi:10.1017/pls.2018.21

Walsh, P. F. (2018). *Intelligence, Biosecurity and Bioterrorism.* London: Springer.

Walsh, P. F. (2021). Transforming the Australian Intelligence Community: Mapping Change, Impact and Challenges. *Intelligence and National Security, 36*(2), 243–259. https://doi.org/10.1080/02684527.2020.1836829

Walsh, P. F. (2022). Securing the Bioeconomy: Exploring the Role of Cyberbiosecurity. In *The Handbook of Security* (pp. 335–355). Cham: Springer International Publishing.

Walsh, P. F., & Bernot, A. (2023). Submission to the 2024 Independent Intelligence Review (13 November). https://researchoutput.csu.edu.au/ws/portalfiles/portal/415490162/Walsh_Bernot_Submission_to_2024_Independent_Intelligence_Review_13Nov.pdf

Walsh, P. F., Ramsay, J., & Bernot, A. (2023). Health Security Intelligence Capabilities Post COVID-19: Resisting the Passive "New Normal" within the Five Eyes. *Intelligence and National Security, 38*(7), 1095–1111.

Wang, L., Shang, L., & Zhang, W. (2023). Human Genome Editing After the "CRISPR Babies": The Double-Pacing Problem and Collaborative Governance. *Journal of Biosafety and Biosecurity*, 5(1), 8–13. doi:10.1016/j.jobb.2022.12.003

Watters, K. E., Kirkpatrick, J., Palmer, M. J., & Koblentz, G. D. (2021). The CRISPR Revolution and Its Potential Impact on Global Health Security. *Pathogens and Global Health*, 115(2), 80–92. doi:10.1080/20477724.2021.1880202

West, R. M. & Gronvall, G. K. (2020). CRISPR Cautions: Biosecurity Implications of Gene Editing. *Perspectives in Biology and Medicine*, 63(1), 73–92. doi:10.1353/pbm.2020.0006

White House (2022a). *National COVID-19 Response Plan*. Washington, DC: White House.

White House (2022b). Executive Order on Advancing Biotechnology and Biomanufacturing Innovation for a Sustainable, Safe and Secure American Bioeconomy. Retrieved from www.whitehouse.gov/briefing-room/presidential-actions/2022/09/12/executive-order-on-advancing-biotechnology-and-biomanufacturing-innovation-for-a-sustainable-safe-and-secure-american-bioeconomy/

WHO (2021). Early-Warning 'Pandemic Hub' Plan Unveiled by WHO's Tedros and Germany's Merkel. Retrieved from https://news.un.org/en/story/2021/05/1091332

Wilson, J. (2017). Signal Recognition During the Emergence of Pandemic Influenza Type A/H1N1: A Commercial Disease Intelligence Unit's Perspective. *Intelligence and National Security*, 32(2), 222–230.

Worobey, M., Levy, J. I., Serrano, L. M., Crits-Christoph, A., Pekar, J. E., Goldstein, S. A., Andersen, K. G. (2022). The Huanan Seafood Wholesale Market in Wuhan Was the Early Epicenter of the COVID-19 pandemic. *Science*, abp8715. doi: 10.1126/science.abp8715

Index

For Product Safety Concerns and Information please contact our EU
representative GPSR@taylorandfrancis.com
Taylor & Francis Verlag GmbH, Kaufingerstraße 24, 80331 München, Germany

www.ingramcontent.com/pod-product-compliance
Lightning Source LLC
Chambersburg PA
CBHW060301220326
41598CB00027B/4195